*Taceant colloquia. Effugiat risus. Hic locus est
ubi mors gaudet succurrere vitae.*

What does the Pathologist say?

FERNANDO VERDÚ

What does the Pathologist say?

Observations on the Methods and Capabilities of Forensic Medicine

FERNANDO VERDÚ

Professor of Legal and Forensic Medicine at the
Universitat de València, Spain

Translators

Terry Kent and Emily Maletin-Kent

Translation of "¿Qué dice el forense? Una curiosa sinopsis de ciertas quisicosas, peculiaridades y técnicas de la medicina legal y forense"

Published by EDITORIALCOMARES, Granada, 2002

Thirteen years later, also... To my dear sons Fernando and Juan Javier.

Writing this book, and numerous other activities, has not stopped me enjoying your company.

Thank you for being as you are

AS A TRIBUTE

This is a translation of the second edition of ¿Qué dice El Forense? The latter was produced with a constraint that could never be overcome. The great authority, the late Professor Gisbert Calabuig, Don Juan Antonio, could not see the original before publication.

He would surely have made some suggestions that, after discussion, I would have inevitably accepted; but I have now taken on his mantle.

From the thirtieth day of May 2000, he has no longer been with us; so we miss his criticism or his approval; but still we have his disciples, his works and our memories.

Many who were privileged to learn from him over many years are yet to see the full effect of it. Therefore, the presence of the Master has not gone - he continues to be with us.

Fernando

PREFACE TO THE SECOND EDITION

The final decision to produce a new edition and not just to reprint was not taken lightly. The first edition was well received by professionals, students and laymen and covered most of the problems in forensic medical investigations. However, there remained outstanding a fundamental aspect of any criminal investigation; the offender.

That 'there is nothing new under the sun,' when introducing the reader to the reality of forensic medicine, is still true. But it continued to irritate me that the reader was not being helped to find the offender. I have therefore decided not to change anything in the original chapters but add an Appendix.

In fact so far as the basic information, there was little to change. Perhaps a few details; for example, when I refer in the introduction to the legal definition of a corpse that, strictly speaking, is no longer valid. In fact, in Spain, after being in force for 21 years, the law on postmortems and associated clinical issues was replaced by a regulation issued by Royal Decree 2070 on 30 December 1999 regulating the obtaining and clinical use of organs from donors and the transplantation of such organs and tissues.

The original definition of brain death has also been modified as has the concept of death by cardiac arrest.

Indeed, the preamble of the cited regulation is an accurate reflection of the significance and contribution of forensic medicine, as a discipline, on the development of the law, it states:

"Scientific and technological developments of recent years in the fields of medicine and biology; in particular as regards the diagnosis of brain death, and preservation and practices of organ transplants, require the updating of the regulations governing such matters ... "

Something else which has transpired, a source of satisfaction for all, is the implementation of the procedures of the Institutes of Legal Medicine in all the Spanish Autonomous Provinces, I am confident that this is right and inevitable. It is a way of working that should benefit everyone; and it largely depends on us to implement it.

In the new Appendix I have tried to collate some of the contributions from forensic science that can identify an offender. As you will see, there are contributions from forensic medicine and wider forensic science, which combine to assist the investigation.

It only remains for me to thank friends and colleagues who have helped me to get to this point. The result is now in your hands.

Fernando

A NECESSARY CLARIFICATION

"Medical Jurisprudence, or Forensic Medicine, is the science concerned with the application of medical knowledge to certain branches of civil and criminal law".

These words come from the eighth edition of "Medical Jurisprudence and Toxicology" by Glaister, published in 1945, and they go back to the first edition of 1902.

But before that date, individuals such as Andrew Duncan Sr. and Jr., William A. Guy, Robert Cowan, and later Sir Sydney Smith and Sir Bernard Spilsbury along with other prominent leading medics highlighted the enormous importance of the science and what potential forensic medicine has to offer for the application of justice.

The work you now have in your hands, thanks to the generosity and efforts of Terry Kent and Emily Maletin-Kent, addresses part of this science: the application of medical and biological knowledge to clarify the circumstances surrounding a death.

Forensic medicine can have many other applications, in addition to explaining causes of death. Because of this and differing legal and policing structures in different parts of the world, the organization of forensic medicine varies. The structure, the titles, and the roles of the various professionals involved in forensic medicine vary from country to country. Even in the English speaking countries we will find words such as 'autopsy' used in the United States and 'post mortem' in the United Kingdom.

One of the key figures in the UK is the Coroner, who is legally, but not necessarily medically, qualified. In the US, Coroners are being replaced by Medical Examiners, who are medically qualified and sometimes legally qualified as well.

Essentially the Coroner is legally responsible for the investigation of the causes of deaths. They can decide, after the initial notification, whether a death can be classified as natural, or accidental, and not require further procedures; or be suspect and require further investigation. Where there is any doubt a Forensic Pathologist will be called upon to carry out the post-mortem to assist the Coroner to reach his final conclusions. Usually in suspicious deaths a Forensic Pathologist will also attend the scene of the death for a preliminary examination of the body and its surroundings.

In the event that a Forensic Pathologist is not available in some jurisdictions a qualified Pathologist may be allowed to carry out the autopsy.

Other medical professionals assisting police investigations are Police Surgeons, who unlike the Coroner, again are medically qualified. They may also, in contrast to the Coroner and the Forensic Pathologist, also work with the living. They will carry out examinations of victims of physical or sexual assault and for example take blood samples when required.

In Spain, you will find, the model is different. There is a so called 'Coroner' but they can handle cases of both living and dead. They can handle the analysis of an assault with a weapon not resulting in death, but also study the body found at the bottom of a swimming pool.

Things are gradually changing with more and more specialization. Meanwhile, the title of this book, ¿Qué dice el Forense? could be translated as a perhaps ...What does the Pathologist say? ... Let us see.

Fernando

P.S: Thank you very, very much, Terry and Emily.

In pursuing their own professions, judges, magistrates, prosecutors, court clerks, lawyers and the police, are often confronted with situations and events, where, for an accurate understanding, they need the help of forensic medicine.

It is not always easy however for them to find clear, understandable and yet rigorous help to facilitate their work.

With the object of helping to fill this gap, Professor Verdú has written a work that I am pleased to present, and which requires no further embellishments.

The author, from among the many things that can be asked of a medical examiner, has selected, an important criminological and legal theme; from the removal of a body, to the procedures of the autopsy, including the external and internal examinations and taking of samples.

He modestly points out that his medical, biological and other scientific observations assist the administration of justice. Information is collected from specialist knowledge and observations performed logically, with common sense and considerable patience.

From these observations the examiner tries to respond, in an appropriate way, to the questions the lawyer, the judge, or the insurance company, etc. ask of him after particular events.

Well, as a layman, moderately interested in the subject, I can assure everyone that the objectives have been achieved. Fernando Verdú has far exceeded the point of getting a squeamish reader, hyper-sensitive, as I am, to flick with ease, almost with delight, through page after page of the various systematic and orderly chapters of this work.

Through reading this I find answer to many of the issues that the discovery of a corpse pose; in such a way that the imponderables may be resolved.

Indeed, through the examples set by the author, and other information he provides, he almost convinces us that we would be able to solve a murder case, albeit that this is not the purpose of the book. Fernando Verdú only intends to explain, in terms understandable to the lawyer or the police, what they can and should do in each case, and what to expect from the medical examiner's opinion, and how they came to their conclusions.

With remarkable realism he shows us the possibilities and limitations of forensic medicine and questions the image of it as an exact science presented in films and novels, and does so with simplicity and humour, modestly downplaying his efforts.

Appearance should not confuse the reader, because this is not a trivial publication, by a dilettante, but rather a mature work, for only after many years of work, many hours of reflection is it possible to "put into words" the wealth of knowledge that has been accrued by teacher Verdú, in such an entertaining and concise way.

For the reasons outlined above, I strongly recommend reading *¿Qué dice el Forense?* 'What does the Pathologist say?

"A very valuable book for professionals who are specialists in this area and equally useful for any students of law or criminology".

Enrique Orts Berenguer
Professor of Criminal Law
Universitat de València

TRANSLATORS' NOTE

We hope that this volume, describing the various aspects, and explaining some of the details, philosphy and history, of forensic medicine will provide some insight to those with a general interest in the subject. It may also help the broad spectrum of people who come across evidence provided by pathologists, police surgeons and medical examiners in their work, to understand the capabilities and limitations of forensic medical examinations. Fernando has treated what can at times be an extremely disturbing subject with a light hearted style which is difficult to bring across in an English language version. Some compromises have also had to be made due to differing termninologies; we hope this does not detract from the overall aims of the book.

There is no straightforward translation of 'Forense' but this term in Spanish describes those trained and skilled in the theoretical and practical skills of investigating deaths, injuries and even mental disorders with particular reference to the administration of justice. In other jurisdictions these may be termed Pathologists, Police Surgeons or Medical Examiners.

Terry Kent and Emily Maletin-Kent

CONTENTS

CHAPTER

1

Introduction

If anything is misunderstood among the many medical specialisms, it is Forensic Medicine. Even those who are the least knowledgeable understand what Cardiology, Rheumatology, Gynecology and so on are; there could be doubts about Stomatology, since as you well know, it does not deal with diseases of the stomach, but the mouth, etc.

However, very few know much about Forensic Medicine. Those few who have some knowledge, including perhaps some of you, are likely to come from one of three distinct groups.

In one of them we find some college students. They may be graduates in medicine, who must include in their undergraduate studies, a subject called Forensic Medicine. Other students who must also pass the medico-legal Rubicon are Graduates of the Diploma in Law and Criminology. Perhaps for the latter this is one of the subjects that should be considered fundamental.

In another group are those we may call legal practitioners, among which are; justices and judges, prosecutors, court clerks, lawyers and other staff serving in the administration of justice. Most of them are highly knowledgeable in this area and, above all, understand its value.

Finally, the last of the groups are all those who, directly or indirectly, have had some contact with the administration of justice as individuals and needed such expertise. Without going into details, it could be as simple a matter as a traffic accident in which they have suffered an injury. They will probably remember that one of the things they would have had to do for a compensation claim was to have examinations by a Medical Examiner until they recovered from the accident.

The reports produced by these professionals serve as a basis for the judges, or magistrates, to subsequently establish compensation. By the way, I think this is the right time to clarify that when we speak of 'El Forense' which directly translated into English is 'The Forensic' we are using careless terminology, as the correct description should be 'Forensic Medical Examiner' or 'Forensic Pathologist'.

'Forensic' here in simple terms means that the doctor or other medical specialist is providing evidence relating to a legal case.

The word 'forensic' derives from the Latin *'forum'*, meaning relating to the activity before the courts, i.e. in Chambers, or at the Forum. In fact, in studies leading to the award of the Degree in Law, there is a subject 'Forensic Practice'. It covers the methods and practices to be observed before the bodies responsible for the Administration of Justice. However, in Spain, it has been customary that when someone says ¿Qué dice el Forense? We all know that we are referring to a medical doctor involved in giving evidence in a court case.

Although, strictly speaking, it could be a linguist with special knowledge of Aramaic, which had been requested by the judicial authorities to clarify the content of a document involved in legal proceedings. The document being written in Aramaic, of course.

Or a fireman, always unmistakable, with his brilliant helmet, fireproof coat, resistant boots and dripping hosepipe, that had to report and tell a Court the best way to put out a fire.

That said I at least consider it necessary to ask the question: What is Forensic Medicine?

To answer this question, no better way than to resort to the definition of my late teacher (*with your permission, Don Juan Antonio*) Professor Gisbert Calabuig, of the Universities of Granada and Valencia, father of Spanish Legal Medicine, and tutor of some of the leading specialists in our discipline. This much admired Teacher of Legal Medicine said *"it is the set of medical and biological knowledge necessary for solving legal problems, both in the practical application of the law and in its development and evolution."*

Without questioning its clarity and justice, to understand the full breadth of this definition one must start by realizing that laws are dictated by norms of social behaviour and customs. These customs are then defined and codified to maintain acceptable social behaviour.

That is, as societies have evolved, it has become necessary to issue new rules and to revise some of the pre-existing laws to adapt to the society and times they are in. Many of these changes have very evident medical connotation, hence the current relationship established between the medicine and justice and, more broadly, with the law.

To try to illustrate this close relationship I'll give an example so that you can see how the very existence of a human being is affected from conception - or even earlier – until long after his death, by legal regulation in which medicine plays a decisive role.

Before the fertilisation that gives rise to a new human being, there may be cases of genetic manipulation. The Spanish Penal Code allows it, if being used to eliminate a disease and prohibits it, among other circumstances, if intending to carry out human cloning experiments.

If we continue with the act of conception, we can not forget that, at present, there are sophisticated medical and surgical techniques to assist reproduction. It may be superfluous to point out that its application is also regulated by specific laws. In addition, non-consensual insemination of women is now criminalized.

After conception, the continued foetal development may depend on regulations, controlled by Laws with regard to elective abortion. It may be recalled that, in Spain, despite having a new Penal code, Article 417 of the repealed act continues in force pending the issue of a new regulation on abortion.

The above applies where there are serious defects in the foetus, or there are risks to the life of the mother. For the abortion to be considered 'not an offence' there must be subsequent appropriate pathological evidence which corresponds to the reports presented by doctors prior to the application for the abortion.

Once the birth has occurred parents will know the legal requirements regarding the registration of the child in the Civil Register. The legislation that requires this, the Law and Civil Registration Regulations, also has considerable medical content.

Putting aside, for the moment, the other times during anyone's life that they will come into contact with various judicial rules and regulations; they eventually reach the moment of death. Usually a doctor, after confirming the death, must issue the obligatory death certificate. This is the document that allows compliance with the regulations for recording the death, in the vast majority of occasions.

However on other occasions the death may have to be established by application of specific procedures when there is the possibility of removing organs for transplanting. It may then be necessary to established brain death.

The indications of death are not then the death certificate, but the symptoms and signs required legally that indicate that life has ceased.

Once death has occurred, we are all familiar with what happens at the end, it is necessary that it is entered into the Register of Deaths, after the death certificate has been issued.

There are other connections between medicine and the law.

If the death has been due to certain causes, some infectious diseases, radioactivity etc. if the family wish to carry out an exhumation to transfer the remains it may not be possible due to regulations imposed by the authorities controlling interment, either local or national.

Actually after death in Spain, bodies are classified into two groups: Group I if death is caused by an infectious or contagious disease, cholera for example, or the action of radioactive materials; and Group II where the death was from another cause.

The former are subject to restrictions on movement, whereas with the latter the transfer only has to meet a minimum of formalities.

As I reflect on the above, the evolution and development of legislation has been directly influenced by medicine, thus fulfilling one of the aspects that were included in the definition of Legal Medicine

It is, in short, something that continuously develops and is in tune with the constant advances in science, which may astonish, or worry, or sometimes scare us.

"and Forensic Medicine?"

Another aspect of our discipline is to be seen as helping the administration of Justice when a specific case must be solved in law, and they need to reach the correct decision with the help of special medical and biological knowledge.

Since the members of the judiciary are only human, and do not have a comprehensive understanding of all aspects of science, they therefore require support from medical professionals who can help them to resolve some cases.

The Spanish National Body of Forensic Doctors, or Pathologists, has its origins in 1855, and I proudly say that I have the honour to be a member.

Forensic Medicine is almost automatically associated with autopsies and these specialists carry out work of great importance despite conditions which are less than ideal and generally with great dedication and deserving greater recognition. Their contributions are actually provided by expertise in very diverse fields; and again, all for the general good of society.

Thus, they are needed when a sexual assault may have been committed; when the abuse of children is suspected; when there has been an accusation of a physical assault; when there has been injury in traffic accidents;

when there is the possibility that there has been driving of vehicles under the influence of alcohol, etc.

This is to say in any situation in which the physical state of a person, both before or after the fact, may have a legal significance. The area of forensic medicine which perhaps is most often publicised, second only to autopsies, is that of forensic psychiatry.

In these cases, in simple terms, the experts have to inform the court about the mental state of a person who, at least apparently, has committed a crime. The psychiatric forensic reports are to guide the courts in making decisions on the criminal responsibility of possible offenders. Forensic psychiatry, however, frequently involves working with victims and witnesses.

The purpose is similar: to report on the mental state of an individual, to facilitate a better judicial decision.

But there is no denying the star activity of the Medical Examiner, or Pathologist, from the popular viewpoint, and it is to the practice of forensic autopsies that this book is dedicated and to explanation of this judicial procedure.

By the way: I doubt it that anyone thinks that justice is about a coach full of court officials pulled by horses. It is simply about processes in the course of the legal proceedings. Actually there is a significant lack of investment in the criminal justice system but not disastrously so.

Autopsies must be carried out, according to our Criminal Laws, in all cases where a person's death occurs in violent or suspicious circumstances. The objectives are essentially to establish the cause of the death and to clarify the possible circumstances resulting in the death. To achieve these objectives we need, in a systematic way, to study the complex collection of data that results from the examination of a corpse, starting right from the moment of recovering the body.

The autopsy continues in three principle stages of forensic procedures. The external examination; the internal examination; and the taking of samples for subsequent analysis. When all the results of these examinations are available the autopsy report, as I indicated earlier, should provide statements on the cause of death and the circumstances surrounding it. It will therefore be the examination of cadavers, forensic pathology, which constitutes the central theme of this volume.

With this first chapter I have attempted to provide a brief overview of the work usually performed by medical examiners but actually there are almost endless possibilities and ramifications.

The development of the science of Forensic Medicine places it between medicine and criminal investigation. However most of us involved in it fully understand that it is not 'police work' as such.

Ours are the scientific, medical, biological or psychological observations, but later we have to make a legal interpretation of the same, with the sole purpose of aiding the better and fairer administration of justice.

After these words of introduction, and emphasizing one or two things, I believe this is the moment to get going. I should say that to cover all the questions in the titles of each chapter I shall occasionally repeat things. I will try however to minimize this and when it is inevitable be as succinct as possible.

Well, let's get down to business.

Let's see:

- *"¿Qué dice el forense?"*,"What does the Pathologist say?"

CHAPTER
2

Sure he's dead?

The first action of a pathologist after receiving a call is to establish that, indeed, what he is going to remove from a scene is a corpse and not a person thought to be dead.

Therefore it must be established that death has occurred. To establish that the Grim Reaper has taken possession of a body, we must look for two major groups of signs.

In one, logically the first, are gathered all the data or evidence derived directly from the termination of the vital functions of life. The other major group consists of the so-called *cadaveric phenomena*. These phenomena begin at the time that death occurs and are irreversible and will progress, evolving with the time after death. As a prelude to the description of these signs, I would make a point.

There are times that injuries to a body are so traumatic that a systematic and comprehensive study of all the vital signs to reach the diagnosis of death is unnecessary. Imagine a traumatic event such as a traffic accident, or occupational injury, in which the direct consequence was the decapitation of the victim.

There is clearly no requirement that a doctor has to investigate whether the vital functions have ceased or not. However, other examination of the body must continue, since some of the following indications may be important - and some of the procedures designed for other purposes, may allow us to draw very important conclusions which we will see in another chapter.

Certainty the diagnosis of death is something that, particularly in the past, has worried many people. This was mainly due to fear of being buried alive - and hearing chilling and harrowing tales of screams and cries coming from churchyards.

Exploiting this fear and obsession is what has enabled certain companies engaged in funeral arrangements, often based in the U.S., to have in their catalogue sophisticated chests or coffins fully equipped with air conditioning installations, food storage and, above all, systems of communication with the outside world.

We need to be sure that procedures are carried out professionally, and without taking short cuts. We can then say that the possibility of being buried alive can be excluded.

It may reassure us that under current legislation in Spain a person cannot be buried less than 24 hours after death has been declared. This is more than enough for some visible, vital, signs of life to be observed and after which, there is no doubt of the passing of life.

Now that you are reassured on this matter let us proceed. Basic continuous operation of these life functions of respiratory, cardiac and neurological activity keep a person alive. This implies that the final cessation of any of these three, will logically confirm death of the individual.

Therefore, to make the diagnosis of death, the pathologist shall verify the existence of certain signs that indicate the complete, absolute and definitive failure, of one or more of these vital functions.

The absence of respiration can be detected by several very different means.

The observation of chest movement or listening to the sounds of the breath in the airways into and out of the lungs, are two of them. However, it should be borne in mind that sometimes, chest movements are almost imperceptible and hence monitoring of lung auscultation can present difficulties. This can be exacerbated by local noise conditions and, perhaps, a doctor's poor hearing!

In the past a number of methods were proposed, or used, that attempted to highlight the absence of breathing. I am quite sure that some will remember seeing them in films.

Detecting the oscillation of the flame of a candle or condensation of the breath on a mirror, by placing these objects close to the mouth and nose, were two of the means used. Note that the chances for misdiagnosis were quite high; high temperatures could prevent condensation on the mirror or, conversely, a draft would make us believe that a corpse was breathing.

Technology has allowed us, for quite some time, to carry out electromyographic recordings. These techniques can detect the existence of any of movement in muscles in the body such as those responsible for breathing. This will considerably reduce the possibility of error. The problem however is transporting such electromyograpic equipment which is not exactly pocket size.

In any case, whatever method we use for this check, monitoring for the absence of spontaneous breathing should be continued for some time so that it can serve as a certain sign of death.

If you, dear reader, hold your breath for a minute or two and then continue breathing, it should not be interpreted as a resurrection, and therefore please, do not go into the street shouting madly "miracle, miracle".

Another of the vital signs of life is the functioning of the heart, the organ that is responsible for pumping the blood around our bodies through the arterial and venous systems. Naturally, as in the previous case, the final cessation of heart function defines the death of the person. A doctor can tell, very easily, if the heart works or not, by cardiac auscultation.

The noises that occur in the heart with each of the, systolic and diastolic movements, are quite noticeable; we only need a stethoscope, a pair of ears, a not excessively noisy environment, care and patience. If there is any doubt, there is always the possibility of performing an electrocardiogram, with which readers will be familiar. But care, patience and prudence, must prevail.

There is another way to check that the heart beats. It is called cardiopuncture, or cardiocentesis, and it can also have a therapeutic use. A needle through the chest is used to puncture the heart.

If the heart is beating, blood will be seen pulsating on the tip of the needle and, if not beating, we can introduce a dose of adrenaline, which can stimulate heart function. This method cannot however be regarded as standard practice to establish the death, although it can save lives.

Of course it is very obvious to everyone that if the heart stops, it will also stop the flow of blood throughout our body. This fact can be detected also very easily. Classical documents of forensic medicine report a traditional technique which was believed to work.

This was to observe the behavior of leeches if they were put in contact with the skin of an apparent corpse. Given its peculiar *Draculian,* feeding system, if blood is not being pumped around the body leeches would fall off. Rather like being served a plate of snails and, after a while you realize they are all empty!

Fortunately, the use of leeches in medicine has disappeared from use so it is unnecessary for the intervention of the Humane Society for Leeches to prevent this inhuman, humiliating and degrading practice.

Before continuing to read, please find a flashlight and a rubber band because we are going to be experimenting. I propose this as a first experiment, throughout the book I may ask again, politely, for this invaluable collaboration.

To conclude the section on signs indicating the cessation of blood circulation here are two anecdotal but more recent methods.

The first is to put a flashlight in, for example, the palm and to observe the light that comes through the back, you can do this with the ear, but you must either have a huge ear or you need a mirror. The reddish hue is only seen in the living body, not a corpse.

Try it and see. I should warn you that in the event that the person you test is of the nobility, the colour perceived will, of course, be blue!

The second and final sign that can be used to demonstrate the existence of peripheral blood circulation looks a lot like child's play. Take a rubber band, if you can find one, they always seem to disappear from the drawer I put mine in. Put it tightly around the middle of a finger and leave it for a few minutes.

If the fingertip begins to look like a fat sausage it is OK, you are alive. Otherwise, I can not explain how you may be reading this book, because you're a corpse; for sure.

Before discussing the indications of death that result from the cessation of neurological function in detail we must remember that both cardiac and respiratory functions can be supplied temporarily by artificial techniques.

There are cases therefore where some of the indicators of death which I have outlined so far cannot be used. Consider, for example, a person who is on a ventilator or who has some form of artificial blood circulation.

They are of course 'breathing', or have blood circulation, so the third life function indicator must be investigated. This is the cessation of neurological functioning. So far the only one for which no effective 'mechanical' replacement has been found.

Similar to the case of the complementary cardio circulatory function. We here make a distinction between the signs derived from the cessation of central neurological functions and the ceasing of peripheral functions, although both are also intimately interrelated.

To explore the cessation of peripheral neurologic function numerous tests have been proposed, with highly variable complexity. One of them is investigating the disappearance, after death, of the ability of muscles to respond to electrical stimulation and contract. The technique is performed approximately as follows: placing a needle into each end of the muscle chosen for investigation and attempting to activate with an electrical current.

In the case of a corpse, the selected muscle will not respond to this electrical stimulation. Actually, this loss of response does not occur at any precise moment, but occurs gradually after death. We will see later that this also occurs with some other observed signs.

Similar to the previous, but more extensive, is the other called transcerebral testing by electric shock. In this case, what is done is to direct the electrical current throughout the body and through brain and their neural connections. This test has the advantage, moreover, that it can serve as a resuscitation technique, as in the case of cardiopunture, or cardiocentesis.

So we have addressed the study of signs that indicate the absence of life in the central neurological system. I question however, precisely, in a legal context, where we will find the best definition of cadaver.

I say this because if we consult the Royal Academy Spanish Language Dictionary (DRAE) it is rather unsatisfactory and tautological.

I refer to the facts that a cadaver, according to DRAE, is a "dead body".

If we seek the original meaning of "body", we see that it is "something that has limited size and produces impression on our senses for qualities which are unique" and finding "dead" defined as "being without life", we could conclude, without doubt according to this definition, that a traffic light, for example, is a 'dead body' or cadaver.

So, as much as we would like a clear definition, I am afraid, the dictionary is of little help here.

Legally the definitions relating to the law regulating the removal of organs from cadavers, for later use in transplants, say that a corpse is "a body in which the vital signs are not detectable for a continuous period of thirty minutes and this state continues over a period of six hours after the initiation of a coma. The absolute loss of consciousness with no brain response to any stimulus, the absence of spontaneous breathing, lack of cephalic reflexes with lack of muscle tone, both eyes dilated and, finally, a flat electroencephalogram demonstrating the vital electrical inactivity of the brain."

With all this we mean that the brain no longer functions; and it will never function again. And if the brain is dead, the person to which it belongs is similarly so.

The above reflects the known current criteria of brain death which in most cases should be confirmed before taking of organs from a donor cadaver to transplant to a recipient in need of an organ.

These criteria are valid provided that the body has not been subjected to the action of drugs that depress the central nervous system or has been found in conditions of very low temperature, or hypothermia.

For very young children requirements are more stringent, since the lack of maturity makes their vital signs different.

Although there are many signs that can be studied more, I will stop here with my description of diagnosing death based on the study and verification of the cessation of vital functions. But remember that we still have to see the signs due to initiation of cadaveric phenomena.

To begin at the beginning, which is often the best way, the first thing to say is that the so called cadaveric phenomena, the changes to a body after death, are considerably influenced by environmental factors. These various signs of death may require longer, or shorter, times to show themselves.

Twenty-four hours after death we will surely find them and, as noted at the beginning of the chapter, the law prevents burials being carried out before this time.

Some of these signs are well known in particular *rigor mortis*, coldness and putrefaction. I will talk more about them in another chapter.

But there are other lesser-know signs which are of considerable value as we shall verify later; if you are still able to continue with the reading of this book,

One is the loss of water from various areas of the body, a fact that was originally called dehydration cadaverous. As I indicated it is a phenomenon much less known by the general public but it is undoubtedly of great forensic value. Among the signs attributable to loss of body fluids, there is one that perhaps may be better known to you. I refer the appearance of the eyes of corpses in that the cornea has lost its transparency, so the appearance is dull. Lifeless.

The livor mortis, post mortem lividity or hydrostasis, is another phenomenon which may be observed, these are a kind of red-blue 'stain' that is visible through the skin and which are caused by a very simple process.

When the heart is functioning, the blood circulates through the arterial and venous system of the body powered by the wonderful operation of the heart as a pump.

At the moment the heart stops, there is no longer this driving force and it is then that the effect of Earth's gravity on the blood, which is no longer in circulation, starts.

The 'livor mortis' occur in those areas of the body that are closest to the ground.

If, for example, the body is lying face down, the livor mortis appear on the face, chest, abdomen, and so on.

Conversely, if the body is hanging by the feet, the aforementioned stains will then be the lower half, i.e. in the head and trunk, and if the corpse is standing, we are likely to get the fright of our lives!

Clearly, if we observe these phenomena on a body, we will be sure that we have a cadaver.

As you see, we now have a large number of objective signs to determine that we have a dead body. What we must do is study them fully and not take anything for granted.

I recommend: attention, patience and prudence. The diagnosis of death is probably the only medical procedure that combines two characteristics: the first is that it is impossible for an error to occur. The second is that this diagnosis may be done by any capable person, without having to become a doctor.

I say it is impossible for an error to occur because, if each and every one of the signs I mentioned in this chapter is observed, the situation is clear. A body that does not breathe for a long time, and where the heart is absolutely quiet, which is cold, rigid with eyes opaque and beginning to expel an unpleasant odor, is a corpse.

A problem can only arise if knowledge of the vital signs to look for is not used properly or there is an incomplete observation. So everyone can diagnose death when these characteristics are shown and you know the cadaver is as dead as a skeleton; even if you are not a doctor.

Anyway I want to convey a message of confidence, security and trust. Making full use of the large number of signs available ensures that, if things are as they should be, today it is absolutely impossible that legal burial could occur of a living person. But, alas, if procedures are bad ......

CHAPTER

3

Who is the *interfecto*[1]?

To start, let me clear up something, mostly for the benefit of clueless reporters, the *'interfecto'* is always a body.

This is one of those words that sometimes we use without knowing exactly their true meaning. Looking at the Spanish dictionary, *'interfecto'* is one who has died violently. Therefore, strictly speaking, we can not speak of the 'interfecto' when the death resulted from natural causes, such as a heart attack or stroke.

---

[1] *Interfecto: Spanish noun meaning someone who has died 'unaturally', this has no simple English equivalent term.*

You will often hear on some news report, something like this: "What did the *'interfecto'* say to him?" Obviously, if the *'interfecto'* answered it would cause some considerable surprise and indignation. This last reaction will be directed, justifiably and naturally, towards the doctor that certified the death.

Well, where were we up to!

For those who carry out autopsies, the identification of a corpse, or of human remains, is an essential part of their forensic examination. This is not to say that achieving a full identification depends exclusively on these experts but many observations made during the postmortem examination make an important contribution to identification. Therefore, those in charge of the investigation should make good use of the pathologist's report.

First of all, do we know exactly what we mean by identity?

As elsewhere, we find many definitions which may help us to get to the real meaning. I am attracted by a clear, concise, definition, whose author may have been a simpleton who could not see further than the end of his nose.

The definition reads: *'Identity is the set of features that makes a person different from others and only the same as themselves'.*

Attempts at identification in forensic medicine may have a far less specific outcome. There are situations when, after investigating the identity of a corpse, all we can do is place it within a group from which it came.

Supposing, as an illustration, that our investigation is focused on two bones, a tibia and fibula, after applying the appropriate techniques, we may conclude, that *'the remains probably belong to a woman, 15 to 20 years old and approximately 160 centimeters tall. Her blood type is B and DNA genetic indicators are consistent with her being Caucasian. In the year prior to death she suffered a broken right tibia that was repaired with a titanium pin'.*

It is obvious that with this information it will be much easier to focus a judicial inquiry into a more limited group of people. When there are hundreds of missing persons, there is then already a high proportion which may be excluded who are men, older women, very tall, very short, have had no injuries, and so on.

As a logical consequence, this can provide great comfort to many families. In contrast, for some others, whose loved ones satisfy these earlier criteria, the anxiety is naturally increased.

The first conclusion we can draw now is that in those cases where the autopsy report begins with the phrase *'This is the body of an unknown man ...'*, the more data that has been collected during the autopsy, the easier subsequent identification will be.

When a national identity document has been found beside the corpse, if the body is sufficiently disfigured as to cast doubt on the identification, we must verify that the fingerprint of the right hand index coincides with that of the national identity files, which I shall come back to later. We must not leave out any detail that we come across, however insignificant it may seem, for in this could be the key to the investigation.

Shall I provide some examples? OK:

The observation of two small reddish depressed areas on the nasal ridge indicates that a person often wore heavy spectacles with a certain shape of support. We should find further similar indication behind the ears. Still with the ears, we find a slightly colouration and something of a callous in the left ear. This would be compatible with regular use of an earphone.

We see strong yellowing of the thumb, index and little finger of his left hand, the nail of the latter slightly blackened. He was a regular smoker holding cigarettes in his left hand and dislodging ash with the little fingernail.

Further research with appropriate techniques may tell us what type of tobacco produced the yellow stains. Many more examples could be given.

But I'd rather you do this exercise; you see, you only need observation and logic.

Regarding the legal and social significance of the identification of bodies, I'll just make a very brief comment. When there is an air or sea accident with multiple victims, it is common to consider those who have died in two separate groups. The everyday explanation is simple. When a person dies and we have his body, he is among the dead, seems logical, does it not? Then you can proceed with all the civil actions arising from death, the execution of the will and inheritance etc.

But when death occurs, or at least is assumed, but the body is not found, or remains are not sufficiently identifiable, that individual has simply disappeared. In these cases, the subsequent civil actions are certainly going to involve a more complicated process.

The final step, if the identification has not taken place and the person continues to be missing, is to urge the judicial authorities to issue a declaration of death. This may allow the family to proceed with the disposal of possessions.

Good, it is time that we put on gloves, protective suit and prepare to identify what we have on 'the table'; a euphemism used to refer to the autopsy table which, incidentally, can be a real wonder, stainless steel of the highest quality, in some medical institutes; or, by contrast, a wooden door on two fruit boxes in some small town mortuaries – you think I am joking?

When it comes to the recently deceased, where decomposition is not very advanced, we apply the same techniques as in the identification of a living person.

I said 'living person' in the last sentence but of course this is a common mistake; 'a person', or 'people', always implies living, a dead person is a corpse. People are always alive the dead are forever dead.

Another common, understandable, and acceptable, mistake, is when we say that a corpse, "has died of xxxx.". Of course, the corpse did not 'die', it was the person that died of xxxx.

Well, back to the identification of the body. Photography is an extremely important procedure, though not infallible. In fact there may be disfigurement which can lead to error. Sometimes you can show a picture of a body of a loved one to some relatives, and they do not identify them. Anyway, good comprehensive photography is essential at any autopsy.

The second method of identification that I will refer to is fingerprints. Everyone knows what they are, but maybe some of you, dear readers may not realise what characteristics they possess that make them useful for the identifying function. I'll try to fill that small, understandable, gap.

Fingerprints start appearing from the third month of foetal development, the skin begins to form very small kinds of folds and associated sunken grooves or creases. These are called the ridges and valleys that make up fingerprints.

The basic shapes taken up like everything in our body are determined by the genetic information but modified by apparently random variations. This makes the variability of shapes and features virtually endless.

Furthermore, the skin has a very considerable resistance, so the study of fingerprints can be done even though the process of disintegration of the corpse by decay has started.

Even with minimal knowledge it is very easy to understand the value of fingerprints for identification work. Without going into great details, the taking of fingerprint impressions allows for two methods of identification.

The first is their comparison with the fingerprint records, whether the criminal records, the prints of the ten fingers of offenders, or the records of the National Document Identity Office. In the latter case, only the fingerprint from the right index finger is recorded from any Spanish citizen who has obtained an official identification document.

There is the other possibility for individuals who are not criminals but have during the incident lost the index finger of their right hand, or the whole hand. The method is to take the fingerprints of the rest of the fingers of the right hand and left hand. We then compare these with fingerprints found on various objects belonging to people who we think could be the unidentified corpse.

Obviously, if a body is found without its hands, fingerprints are about as useful for the identification as a bicycle without wheels is to go for a pleasant ride on a quiet, cool spring morning; or at any other time of year.

Other unique identifiers are specific personal features. These are characteristics, or peculiarities, that can be observed on bodies and, occasionally, can provide definitive information to establish identity.

Among the special features I would emphasize first is the presence of physical defects. Thus, one leg shorter than the other, the presence of six digits on a hand or foot, the presence of a cleft palate, etc. are data that should also be recorded if seen during an autopsy. This should be done automatically even if at this initial stage identification is not expected to be a problem.

A second group of characteristics that should not be overlooked, for the considerable value that they can bring, is the presence of scars. These may be the permanent signs of surgical incisions, or where as the result of an accident, permanent scarring has been left.

Scars are of different value and of course an appendectomy scar is different to one from heart surgery. One aspect that must never be overlooked is the possibility that a scar, with particular characteristics, has been changed by subsequent surgery, with the object of 'obscuring' its previous appearance.

Finally I note that sometimes the scars are not as easily detected as they were, due mainly to the great advances in plastic and reconstructive surgery. It is therefore advisable to examine the body with the help of some light source that favors the perception of the scar tissue, such as ultraviolet light. The color differences between normal and damaged areas then can become much more evident.

Other identifying signs are tattoos that are as common now as in the past, although they are restricted to certain limited social groups. They continue to be of inestimable value; especially when the tattoo consists of the full names of the deceased along with their National Identity Number!

As in the case of scars, tattoos may also be modified by subsequent interventions. In this way the so characteristic and common

Amor (Love)

De (of)

Madre (Mother)

can easily become a surprising

Amoralidad

(Debauchery)

Desenfreno

(Rampage)

Desmadre (Chaos)

There are other identifying features; again, I invite you to exercise your imagination. For example, if you have a brother who loves fishing, examine his teeth and you will see that he probably has a defect in the cutting edge one of his incisors. This defect is caused by a nasty habit of cutting the line with his teeth, rather than with a suitable instrument.

If death has occurred some time ago and putrefaction is already manifest it will cause problems as there are major changes in the external appearance of the body. Now the recognition and identification can become much more difficult. But we should not forget that some characteristics that we have already studied may remain recognizable for some time. Such is the case with fingerprints or tattoos.

Let us continue further; now for the situation when what we are examining is no longer a corpse, strictly speaking, but some human remains.

When we have a complete skeleton to study the procedure is simpler, the information obtained may be sufficient to establish, with a high degree of reliability, sex, age and race.

This is done by exploiting the morphological data from a large number of skeletal elements: for example, the skull of a man and a woman are different; the bones of a 20 year old are not the same as a 75 year old etc.

Also, studying bones can determine the approximate time of death. This is done by assessing the amount of bone mineral components in relation to its organic fatty components.

The cause of death is another problem that may possibly be resolved. Indications can be obtained, for example, by the existence of broken bones caused by gun shots or by the detection of heavy metals such as lead, which tend to accumulate in the bones.

We should also establish whether there are artificial implants in the bones, such as prostheses, metal plates or pins, which can become very important elements of individual identification. I will take up all these aspects in slightly more detail in other chapters of the book.

When we turn our attention to the skull of course we have some important evidence to assist the judiciarl identification. The aspect that is of most interest for identification purposes is forensic odontology of the teeth; but we should not ignore the palate, it is perhaps less well known that this is also of value.

The palate, whilst coping with the bones of a fish, or crunching in some tasty crust of bread may serve to assist in identification. Touch your palate now and notice two things. One, occasionally that it will tickle. The other that is has features, shapes and characteristics; and every one develops differently.

The explanation, much like I have given above for fingerprints, is that the palate adopts a particular morphology from very early in the fetal life and remains unchanged throughout our life. Also similar to the fingerprints is that its bony nature resists the rapid decay suffered by soft tissue.

With regard to the study of the teeth, jaws and associated parts, there is now much greater awareness and many publications so I will only mention two things. If it is individual parts, or rather fragments of jaws, the two important things which can be reliably predicted are sex and height.

When you can study the maxilla and mandible, the confidence of identifications can be as accurate as fingerprints. This is because they can combine three types of characteristics: the various forms of each of the teeth, the diseases that can affect them and, finally, the remedial dental procedures that have been applied to treat them.

These studies are used most often in cases of major disasters that are accompanied by fire. In these situations, the refractory nature of teeth and bones make these, at times, the only reliable data identifiers.

However, their potential use is restricted by something very obvious. If there is nothing to compare them with their value is zero.

Remember that in the case of fingerprints taken from cadavers, we must compare them, for example, with existing records. Unfortunately it is rare to find such a complete dental record. In the case of aircraft accidents, there is normally a passenger list. In these cases, you must ask the families of the missing about their visits to dentists. If these consultations are regular, you contact the dentist who can provide the dental records necessary to help the identification.

The final biological identifiers to which I will refer are blood grouping and deoxyribonucleic acid, or DNA. It is prophetic that only one letter differentiates two such important instruments of identification as the DNI, The Spanish Document of National Identity, and DNA. In a few years, when the human genetic map is completed, we will be able to talk of DNAI, i.e. deoxyribonucleic acid identity.

The techniques used for analysis are very complex and beyond the scope of this book but DNA analysis may be carried out on body parts as diverse as blood, hair, bones, flesh, teeth, skin, etc., making it virtually impossible to find human remains where it cannot be applied.

If a full DNA typing is achieved it is not possible to confuse the identity of a person with anyone else except in the case of identical (monozygotic) twins. These individuals have developed from the fertilization of a single egg with a single sperm, so their genetic material is absolutely identical.

However, it appears that studies suggest the existence of two differentiating characters for monozygotic twins. The first is the way in which the brain neurons establish their interconnections. The second is the patterns of the ridges on the fingers, the fingerprints, which are different. So such individuals could be distinguished by examining their fingerprints.

Anyway, I am seized by a doubt. If all of our characteristics are determined by the molecules of DNA: what reason is there for personality differences to exist?

Environmental influences? Genetic mistakes? Time will tell.

Leaving the strictly medical field one should take account of what we might call extrinsic identifying elements.

Rings, bracelets, watches, chains, necklaces, earrings, handbags, cards and other personal items must be documented with care, as they may also have a great significance for the conclusion of the investigation. Thus, in the case of a plane crash, preceded by an explosion, it is possible that there may be body parts such as hands, with a ring, or an ear with an earring.

What you must never do is separate the body part from the jewelry: This act can make a person pass from the group of known dead to the missing group, with all the problematic consequences that this implies.

I will conclude this brief, but I think illustrative, foray into the identification techniques used in the forensic field, with a curious reference. In aviation accidents there are two bodies that are generally easily identified: those belonging to the pilot and copilot.

This relative ease is based on the study of stomach contents as they are two people that because of the responsibility of their job usually do not eat the same food. This prevents any food poisoning affecting them both.

Well, now we know that *'so and so'* is dead, we will continue to investigate. We will see in the next chapter, that you can forget the idea that the work of a medical examiner is waving a magic wand.

Neither is it a crystal ball or tarot cards or a Ouija board ...

Only science, patience and care. Observation and logic.

CHAPTER
4

When did they die?

I start this fourth chapter with another question which the Medical Examiner must answer at the completion of a judicial autopsy. Determining as accurately as possible the time of death of a person is one of the major daily challenges presented to the Medical Examiner or Pathologist.

In fact, some of the great masters of the discipline have considered this to be an unattainable goal. This has not prevented much research having been carried out and some being still underway with the objective of achieving greater accuracy over the time when the transition between life and death has occurred.

Perhaps we should remember the proverb "Do not say it is impossible". Only say: *"It has not yet been done."*

This seems like a Chinese proverb, but actually it is Japanese.

Well, despite this, we still see in films the scene when, after coming across a corpse, a man, usually about fifty or sixty years of age, generally in a black coat and a hat or bald with glasses, after looking at the corpse, says: "He died about two hours ago."

As I always tell my students, that is absolutely and completely wrong; actually what I usually say is that *" it is soul destroying to hear such nonsense".* The problem, as we will have the opportunity to see, is much, much, more complicated than that.

I will try to show why it is so important to determine the time of death with three or four examples. By the way, if some of you are not convinced, let me know, and I will send you five or six more examples.

When we talk about criminal activities no one would deny the need to know the time of death. This will enable a starting point to be established to help criminal investigations, for instance, in identifying the body of someone who has disappeared, or that the alibi of a particular person is accepted as proving their innocence, or not.

Another relevant and very important aspect of criminal law is the statute of limitations. The Penal Code states, amongst other things, that for crimes with potential maximum sentences of 15 or more years the statute of limitations is 20 years starting from the time the offence was committed.

Establishing when a murder occurred therefore has important consequences. As can be seen, there are times when the judiciary face extremely difficult problems.

In inheritance issues time of death may also have a huge impact: for example that of a childless marriage, but both partners having siblings and parents.

If both spouses die without witnesses to the time of death, three different situations may arise.

If it is established that the woman died before the husband, he is the direct legal heir and owner, but not for long, of the property of his wife. On his death soon after the biggest beneficiaries will be the relatives of man.

If instead it is determined that the husband was the first to die, applying a similar reasoning, the family of the woman will be more fortunate.

Finally, if it is established that both died at the same time there is no transfer of property between the husband and wife to their respective families so that distribution may be otherwise decided.

The civil Spanish Code indicates that: "If there is doubt which of them has died first, unless it can be proved by the claimant; they are presumed to have died at the same time and the transmission of rights does not take place from one to the other". As you can see this is a real 'Judgement of Solomon' situation, in which the so-called burden of proof is on the party seeking to make a profit.

The last example I will talk about is related to life insurance.

In a case of accidental death, the pathologist had to try to establish the time of death, before or after midnight on the night of a given day. The problem arose because at midnight that day, a life insurance policy that the deceased had taken out with 'The Magpie Life Insurance Company' expired.

If, ultimately, the medical examiner states that death has occurred after midnight, the deceased is no longer protected by this important life insurance, which he had arranged to meet the needs of his family.

As on other occasions throughout the book, the case is real, like life itself. But, of course, the name of the insurance company is totally fictitious and any resemblance to a real company must be considered to be coincidental.

As I said a few paragraphs earlier, to define the time of death, is certainly difficult.

The methodology used to determine this is to follow the general scheme advocated by classical Forensic Medicine; dealing first with a case concerned a fresh corpse and then with the older corpses and skeletal remains.

Before we start discussing the subject we have to understand the phenomena of death and we need to know the cause of death. Please be logical.

Broadly speaking, we all know that death is the absence of life. However, the fact that a person dies, does not mean that absolutely all the cells will die at the same time. Do not think that death is something akin to the action of a switch controlling the electric current reaching a light bulb and only has two positions: on or off, life or death.

Following the electrical analogy, it is closer to the action of a rheostat, which as you know, is a device that allows you to vary the amount of current, which passes through a bulb which then provides various intensities of illumination. This mechanism can move from the position of on to off; life-death; gradually, little by little.

Seeing things overall, when a fatal accident occurs, the person as whole, body and soul, dies. But, in isolation, we can find various types of cells that still show signs of activity. They even 'live' and will be gradually, progressively, lost.

Thus, when one is considering a fresh corpse one can use these effects to establish the time of death. Furthermore, and fundamentally, we will also utilize the study of cadaveric phenomena, which I introduced in the previous chapter.

Let us see how we can adjust these and how difficult the task is. Regarding the observation of the time when death occurs in different cell groups, there have been numerous research papers but of course we can only consider some examples here.

Most experiments are conducted in highly controlled laboratory conditions; their subsequent application in forensic practice is not so easy.

If we are studying the body of a man, we can benefit from, for example, the study of the mobility of sperm. It has been shown experimentally that sperm are able to continue moving up to 36 hours after a man's death.

To study them, take samples from the seminal vesicles and observe them with a microscope.

Clearly, if a microscope is not used, this test could not be effective, comparable only to trying to thread a fine needle in a dark tunnel, blindfolded and wearing gloves.

Another aspect that may be used to try to resolve the problem is the present state of digestion of food found inside the body.

To do this we need to know the time the last meal has been eaten and then look at what stage of digestion the various components of the meal are in.

Rice, chickpeas, fish and meat, for example, have different digestion times, so once again, the coroner must seek advice from other experts.

Another fact that has been studied to establish the time of death, has been the growth of beard hairs. They grow about half a millimeter a day and it is known to be a process that stops at the moment of death. If it can be found out when a man shaved last, it should be possible to determine the time of death, by measurement of the length attained by the hair.

The use of this technique has been reduced in recent decades because now, the vast majority of men are not shaved in a barbershop, something which years ago, was widespread.

However, it may be possible to learn from the family or neighbours, by noises heard or any other means, information about this last shave; and the medical examiner can use this wisely.

Another group of useful signs which are relevant to the study of time of death I remind you of are, dehydration, cooling, rigidity and livor mortis. Again we must say that they all go through different phases and the object of the Medical Examiner must be determine precisely at what stages they have reached. This is the best way to extract the maximum possible forensic value. We shall consider each of them.

The dehydration mortis will allow us to approximate the time of death by examination, for example, of the transparency of the front of the eye, i.e. the cornea, which I have previously mentioned as a sign of death.

This area of the eye will lose water very quickly, so about an hour after death, the cornea loses its normal transparency.

But allowance must be made for different rates if the body has remained with eyes open or closed, since in the former case, dehydration is much faster. Logical, of course.

As a result of the loss of fluids from the eye, this structure gradually collapses and becomes softer. The intra-ocular pressure in the eyeball may actually be measured quantitatively using a device called an eye tonometer.

A crude way to establish this loss of fluid is by pressing the eyeball lightly with the fingertips.

The cadaverous livor mortis, those coloured spots that form on the skin, when the heart stops working, can offer valuable information, because we know the approximate rate of development.

Thus, they begin to be formed about forty-five minutes after the death and are considered to be completely extended and set, that is to say they no longer disappear with pressure, after about twenty hours. The extent of the spread of the livor mortis and making them disappear by finger pressure are the two elements that must be considered.

Recently we have tried to use a device that 'measures' the intensity of livor mortis through the skin, although results are not very reliable; but everything will come eventually.

The rigidity of corpses, another of these useful phenomena, also takes place over a specific timeline.

Everyone knows that after the death of a person, two of the first things to do are: closing the eyes and mouth otherwise we risk that after a short time, they will remain open because of the effect of rigor mortis. The muscles of the body, after a complete initial relaxation, will tighten up during the first phase. Then they stay strongly contracted for some time then eventually relax completely.

If we know which of the three phases the rigidity of the body is in, we also know approximately when death has occurred.

Finally, the stage of the cooling of a corpse also provides an invaluable aid.

This phenomenon occurs because inside the body there are no longer the vital processes, which are accompanied by the production of heat, a fact that helps keep our average temperature in the region of thirty-seven degrees centigrade.

At the time death occurs a body usually begins to lose heat and tends to equilibrate to the ambient temperature. Of course, as you realise, patient reader, in the event that the ambient temperature is over thirty-seven degrees, the body does not cool it is heated eventually to the temperature of the environment.

For the most reliable data we measure the temperatures inside the body, either in the rectal or vaginal cavity; or performing an abdominal incision where we can insert a special thermometer to measure 'core body temperature'. However, you can get a first impression by touching the body.

These various indicators exhibit considerable variations and are modified by a number of factors which the expert has to evaluate. The constitution of the body, the existence of previous diseases, the cause of death, weather conditions etc. are just some of them.

Only after considering all of the various indicators can we give an answer, which may not be very accurate, but hopefully may be sufficient to answer the original question.

One word of caution, assessing the progress of cadaveric phenomena should always be taken in two stages. The first time should be at the crime scene, the second time should be several hours later when the body is at the mortuary. The comparison of these observations is invaluable.

But obviously these techniques can only be used if death has occurred fairly recently. What we generally call recent corpses. For less recent corpses, these phenomena are of no use and therefore, we avail ourselves of other sources of information.

I now warn those less hardy spirits. I will talk about the putrefaction of corpses; but try to be gentle and avoid unpleasant references. And I hope that the Editor does not fulfill his threat of using odours to impregnate these pages. Finally, as we say, it is time, forewarned is forearmed. It is well known by all that living organisms undergo decay processes after death and of course, we people are no exception. After life there are a series of physical and chemical changes in our body so that, after many years, it is true that the "Dust Thou Art, and Unto Dust Shalt Thou Return"

If we study a corpse at some point, using a logical methodology we will be able to work out when death has occurred by the state of decomposition it has reached. Elsewhere I will talk a little more extensively about the putrefaction but in advance of that, briefly, I will say that the process of putrefaction goes through four phases.

The first one is called *chromatic,* and there are changes in the color of the body surface. This begins about twenty-four hours after death, with the onset of the *abdominal green spot.*

The second phase is *emphysematous,* or *bloating,* characterized by the formation of gases inside the body from bacteria. It is evident about three days after death.

In the third phase, called *liquefaction* stage, there is the breakdown of the soft tissues, which are losing their original form and shape and collapsing into a sort of amorphous mass, which has a sticky and oily touch. Which by the way: it is very unpleasant.

The fourth phase is the *skeleton,* and is the most persistent of all. This involves the complete disappearance of all soft tissues, viscera and muscles, and more resistant tissue, such as tendons and cartilage. Even after the body is reduced to a mere skeleton, changes occur which consist mainly in the disappearance of the fatty elements within the bone and demineralization. As someone said: "In a hundred years, everyone is bald".

There are many variables involved. Environmental factors such as temperature and ventilation; personal factors such as nutrition; and pathological infection can all affect the rate of decomposition.

By examining these factors we can establish approximately, the time since death whether days, months or years but as on many other occasions, we must be cautious in our conclusions. You see, these things are not simple. In every case we should collect the largest possible number of observations and amount of data so that the conclusion regarding the time of death is consistent with all aspects of our observations of the body.

We must never forget that on this conclusion many very important decisions may depend. As I said at the start, the bald expert with glasses and a black coat from the films is strictly fantasy.

And we have no magic wand!

CHAPTER
5

When they did the injuries occur?

One of the difficult challenges that we have in forensic practice is when have to solve the problem presented in this chapter title. During the autopsy we must find out if injuries which have been found on the body occurred before or after death. Fortunately this is not a situation that arises very often, but when it does occur it is often of great importance. I will try to explain this in the best possible way by illustrating with some examples.

Suppose you see a corpse in a pile of rubble resulting from the collapse of a building after a fire. Logically, to determine exactly the course of events, we must find out when events, and the injuries that we can see, occurred. Probably some of them have occurred while the person was still alive and others, such as those from the collapse, when they where dead. But it could be that the person was dead when the fire started.

In this second case, none of the injuries will have occurred while the person was alive.

Have they been murdered?

Have they committed suicide?

Has it simply been an accident?

Please be patient, because these issues, and their respective answers, belong to another chapter of the booklet.

Another example. A construction worker falls from some height and apparently dies as a result of injuries sustained when hitting the ground. We cannot however rule out that the death may have occurred whilst on the scaffold. Imagine, in this second scenario, that he suffered a heart attack and then fell to the ground.

Finding a corpse at sea, with a major wound in the head, opens up a range of possibilities as to how the death occurred. One of them might be just suffering a fainting spell while bathing and then, after drowning has been hit by a boat. As you can imagine there are many more possible scenarios: a body left in the middle of a road, the corpse of a hanged man, the driver of a car dying in a traffic accident, the body of a walker hit by a train, etc.

But there is a common factor to all these types of cases. The evidence provided from the forensic examination of the event may change, very substantialy; the path the rest of the investigation will take. Considering these issues one realizes the considerable importance to society of the work of the medical examiners. Unfortunately this is not widely recognized and still less appreciated.

Before embarking on a study of the factors that can help us to solve the problem, we should see in what circumstances, injuries can occur. The renowned expert in forensic medicine and lecturer, Thoinot, classified injuries that could occur after death. He did it according to their origin and noted that initially they could be either accidental or deliberate. Those which are simply accidental can be categorized into four major groups.

The first includes all those 'injuries' that are produced by wild life that are common when the body, for example, remains for some time out in the open, immersed in the sea or buried in a shallow grave. Marine, terrestrial and aerial predators are attracted by a food source such as a dead body and can cause considerable destruction, both externally and internally.

A second type is when wounds on the body under consideration are the result of some mechanical action after death such as the propeller of a boat. Indeed, readers will recall the previously discussed head injury of the poor man who had passed out and drowned. Or the blows that can result if a dead body is dumped on a road; the latter is not too uncommon in practice. Everyone has heard that there are drivers, murderers really, who, after running down a person, leave the scene. Soon after, another driver stops his vehicle and alerts the local, highway or state police.

The accident investigation becomes obviously vitally important; so that we do not attribute accountability to someone who has done a humanitarian act. Although it may be a humanitarian act; according to the law in many countries, stopping and reporting is actually obligatory.

The third group includes all those 'injuries' that may occur in the course of the practice of autopsy. These are usually less problematic because the medical examiner must conduct a thorough external examination of the corpse, recording verbally and graphically what he sees prior to making the internal examination.

That way, when they proceed to the opening of the body cavities, the medical examiner, knows whether a particular injury may have been caused by his procedures or, conversely, was caused by something else.

The last group of post-death injuries includes those wounds that may have resulted from extreme pain at the time of death. I can give two examples. One is the existence of a contusion on the head of the corpse of a woman. An autopsy may show that she suffered a major cerebral haemorrhage and, losing her balance, she fell to the floor.

Traumatic injuries can also be found on the arms and legs of a hanged man in convulsions before death by certain types of asphyxiation, due to impact with nearby objects; more about this elsewhere.

There are two other types of post-death injuries resulting from intentional acts, which are classified by

Thoinot as those of medical origin and those of criminal origin.

Of the former, the most common today, are injuries to the sternum or the rib cage caused by attempts at resuscitation. These are usually performed in cases of sudden death. The most striking are those produced by mechanical resuscitators.

The presence of these and correctly noting them can demonstrate that resuscitation procedures have been conducted with appropriate strength and persistence. Indicating that failure to resuscitate has not been due to medical neglect, but to an unrecoverable situation.

Thoinot's post-fatal injuries of criminal origin may have been carried out for various reasons. Sometimes the intention is to disfigure the body and thereby hamper criminal investigations. A good example is of beheading and the amputation of the fingers of a body.

In other cases, the injuries found are the expression of the disturbed mind of the offender, who has sought revenge on the body. We cannot use the term 'torture' if the injuries were inflicted after death; torture is causing pain and suffering to a living person. It is therefore important to establish when injuries have occurred since, if they were alive at the time of the injuries there would be the additional criminal accusation of torture. However, if they were already dead this does not apply.

Finally, there are cases where what the perpetrator intends is for the injuries to conceal the signs of a crime. For example, they kill a person by whatever means and subsequently set fire to the location, a house or a car, or the dead body is placed on railroad tracks for it to be 'knocked down' by the next train.

Now, after all the necessary preparations, gloves, gown, hat and mask, to work!

We can use many signs and methods to find out whether the injuries occurred before or after death. But before going into the detail of the same, I remember writing a few pages ago, that the passage between life and death is not instantaneous, but occurs progressively.

I said there that the process of dying will affect different tissues depending on their nature; in effect, what the power switch and rheostat do in relation to the amount of light produced by a lamp. If we consider this and think logically, a body will respond very differently to an injury if inflicted whilst it is alive, that is, with all the body function running at full capacity; than if inflicted after death.

As death is a transitive phenomenon the reaction to any injury the victim receives will depend on the state of the body's response system at the time of the attack. Some of the signs and techniques we use allow us to identify relatively easily, wounds that have occurred at a time significantly different from the death of the individual, either before or after. Some techniques however are much more complex in their implementation, but may allow us to distinguish if injuries occurred shortly before or shortly after death.

First there is the visual appearance of the injury we are studying. To understand it better, imagine that this is a wound on a finger, for example, by a knife. As usual I appeal to the rich experience of the reader. Please think about the last time you cut yourself, while trying to prepare a sandwich, and answer my questions below honestly.

Did it begin to bleed almost immediately?

While looking for the antiseptic, did blood keep flowing? Did it take a while to clean the coagulated blood stuck to the skin around the wound?

For some hours, did you notice some pain in the injured finger and, taking off the dressing, were the edges of the wound a little inflamed and red?

If you answered yes to all questions is an indisputable fact that when you cut yourself; you were alive!

I have given this example to highlight the things that happen: bleeding, blood clotting and inflammation are characteristic features of a living organism, in which the defense systems are working properly.

In the case of a fracture in an arm by a severe trauma, the basis of diagnosis is similar. In the region of the skin over the site of the injury we will find an intense hematoma and in the center of the fracture there will be a hemorrhage, this is in the case of having occurred to a living person.

If, however, these injuries happened to a corpse you would not find any of these signs.

When instead of a wound there is an abrasion, such as a scratch or scrape against the ground, we also see the presence of typical signs of life, in these cases there is the formation of a scab. This is also indicative of the existence of vital defense system characteristics.

As I said before, this information will help us to differentiate between whether an injury has occurred well before or after the time of death. In the majority of cases it allows us to reach a valid conclusion for the developing investigation.

When we need more accuracy, or the data that we have obtained by the visual examination are not sufficient, we are forced to resort to laboratory techniques. They are certainly more accurate, but have the disadvantage of being far more complex.

One that can be commonly used is the study of some characteristics of leukocytes, or white blood cells, that we will find at the site where an injury has occurred. As you know, leukocytes are cells that are responsible for defending the body in various circumstances. At the time an injury occurs, there is a 'demand' which has the immediate effect that leukocytes, white cells, come to the place where the trauma has occurred with a two objectives.

One mission is to eliminate the remnants of tissue that were damaged, the other is to establish a defense against possible infections. As you may have guessed, this occurs in life, but when the injury occurs after death, there is no such defensive reaction. The leukocytes do not react, 'their role is over'. Therefore study of the injured area, using appropriate microscopic techniques, can prove very valuable.

Another technique that can be used is based on the regenerative capacity of tissues. When an injury occurs very quickly small blood vessels that have been cut react and begin to rebuild the original structure in order to keep the blood flow in the part of the body they supply.

As you can see, nature also has an 'Emergency Plumbing Service' working with startling speed. Again, this is a phenomenon that only occurs in living organisms and its absence in an injury may be a key indication that the assault occurred after death.

Further development of this technique, investigating the enzymes involved, may provide invaluable additional information. Enzymes are substances that are distributed throughout our bodies and involved in virtually all living processes that keep our bodies functioning properly. Precisely because of this characteristic of almost universal intermediary action it has been thought that they could be studied to see how they change when an injury in the organism occurs. In simple terms, I will briefly explain the basis of their use.

In our skin there are various substances that, whenever an injury occurs, change from their normal activity. With various different roles they go to work quickly to repair the damage caused. The different types of enzyme will increase their activity in various parts of the wound and its vicinity depending on their nature.

For example, if there has been a contusion on the right eyebrow, as a result of a severe blow with a stick, you will find two areas with different activities going on. In areas of irreparably damaged tissue there will be an increase in the activity of enzymes that remove dead cells and clean the area in preparation for reconstructing new tissue. In other areas, where the tissue is recoverable, the enzymes that increase their activity will be those with immediate remedial functions.

On this basis, it is obvious that if a wound is inflicted on a dead body, there is no capacity to react, the enzymes are not going to waste time getting to work. So they become 'drifters' like the leukocytes referred to previously. As you can imagine, what I have just said is an oversimplification of a complex process that is also influenced by many factors, but I think as an illustration it is valid.

Establishing whether a wound found on a body has occurred in life or after death may be possible by studying other aspects of our bodies instead of enzymes; but in most cases these new methods are difficult to apply.

I indicated a little while ago that, in most cases, good observation of the morphology of the lesions provides sufficient data to solve the problems that may have arisen. You laymen could also find the answer through good observation. Imagine that you come across a person, seated in a chair, who has an injury on a cheekbone.

If asked, casually, "Hey, when did you hurt yourself?" if he responds, there is no doubt; one can say with absolute certainty that the wound is on someone who is alive.

And without the aid of forensic medicine!

In the event that no answer is heard there can be several causes: deafness, muteness, rudeness, inattention, simple contempt, loss of consciousness, or perhaps because he is dead. Only in the latter case may questions arise that we may attempt to solve by forensic medical techniques.

But I remind you that you cannot always provide an answer, even when every possible technique has been applied.

CHAPTER
6

What was the Cause of Death?

Before setting out the means by which a coroner can establish the cause of death of a person it is appropriate, briefly, to consider in what ways fate can send us to eternity. Traditionally, death mechanisms have been divided into two groups: the so-called direct and indirect mechanisms respectively.

There are what may be termed 'direct death' mechanisms, which can occur in less time than it would take the victim to untie his shoelaces. A typical example of a direct mechanism of death is the destruction of vital brain functions in the skull by a 6 ton weight falling onto the head of a person.

However in cases where death has occurred by a mechanism described as indirect, the initial injury is only a preliminary but crucial step. It initiates a variable length chain, or series, of events which pathologically result in the death of the individual. Here I could give you numerous examples but this might be clumsy and unnecessary so I will give only one which I am sure you will recognize.

Pricking a finger with a nail, in most cases, is something that is not of great importance. But such incidents often cause some concern as we all know that, if the nail is contaminated, it could trigger a deadly tetanus infection.

That would be an indirect mechanism responsible for the death that could be clearly demonstrated. Well, death by direct or indirect mechanisms can result from many types of incident. Restrictions of space prevent me from developing this chapter at length, so I will only speak of some of the methods capable of killing. What is needed is a meticulous study of any injuries, changes and signs on the body caused by an attack. That is the only secret.

First I will discuss the types of contusion which are perhaps the ones that appear most frequently and in many very different circumstances. When you are told, or a medical certificate states that a person has suffered bruising; do not imagine that it is necessarily so clear and simple. To record things properly much more specific detail is necessary.

It's like when we ask "what have you eaten?" and the reply is: "rice".

Rice, yes but what form of rice was it: in seafood paella?, chicken and rabbit paella?, black rice?, white rice?, baked rice? with beans and cod? with mushrooms? with chards? with marsh rats? ,....

You will already have realised that bruises are a group of lesions with a wide range of forms.

We all understand that hitting someone with a fist is not the same as hitting them with an iron bar. In both cases we are going to cause bruising, but in the case of the fist, it is more likely that we cause a darkening or reddening of the skin. While with an iron bar we can also cause a darkening or reddening of the skin but if we have used sufficient force we can break the skin, which would be called a contusion, and in addition cause the fracture of a bone under the area that we struck.

There are times when we find several bruises on a corpse. From their detailed study we can obtain a considerable amount of data to successfully assist the coroner with his objectives; however, as previously indicated do not expect miracles.

As an example on the back of a body we find an ecchymosis, a bruise, that has an elongated shape, with a length of ten centimetres and a width of one centimetre. From that you can only establish that, at some time, there has been a violent contact between a fairly hard instrument which caused the bruising and the body of the victim.

But we cannot establish the nature of that instrument. It may be either a stick, like a club, or the edge of a door, in fact any object, or any part of a structure, which is ten centimeters long and one centimetre wide or so.

However, it will be possible to answer other questions. If a particular instrument is produced as evidence at trial, could this produce that particular injury? Imagine that the incriminating instrument is a steel ball of 15 centimetres diameter and answer this last question yourself.

Another very useful fact is that by examining the bruises we can establish, quite accurately, when the blows were struck. As on many other occasions, the knowledge we apply is nothing very special, and most people know it. Indeed, it is well known that when we strike somewhere on the body we see bruising, at first the area is red and then it changes color. As days go by it becomes successively, blackish-blue, green, and yellow and then finally it disappears.

These color variations are due to changes that occur in the haemoglobin in the blood that form the haematoma and it suffers a decomposition process in which the colors progressively appear. There are two exceptions to this trend in bruises. These are cases where the injury, and the consequent flow of blood to the tissues, has been to a finger or toe nail, or an eye.

I will explain about the nails; do you remember the times when, playing football, instead of skillfully kicking the ball you hit the ground with the same force but rather clumsily, one might say. When I got home I would examine the affected finger and under the nail and see a blackish area. Remember this area moves toward the finger tip with nail growth and disappears with practically no change of color.

Since it is perfectly acceptable that some readers have not played football, you may not have understood what I said in the previous paragraph. To cover that possibility, I would give the example of the hammer and nail. It would go something like this; "do you remember that time when trying to drive a nail, instead of hitting the nail, with such strength and expertise, you hit your finger?" The rest of the text is as before. If you have not played football and also have never hammered a nail, don't bother. Just ask some 'practical' friend what happens!

One other class of implements which can cause injury or kill is referred to as edged weapons. Traditionally this name is given to weapons that are sharp, or have a point, components that will injury. Usually the blades are made of steel, although some training weapons are made of poorer quality iron without a sharp edge.

Before discussing some of the characteristics of this type of injury we need to know something about the structure of skin, as this will allow us to understand better how they occur. You know that in the skin, among other things, there are two types of fibers; collagen, which has no elasticity and which when stretched, breaks. The other fibers are elastic, and allow a degree of stretching, but if excessive force is applied these will also break. Well, edged weapons, of which there are four major groups, act by altering these fibre structures and therefore the appearance of the wounds will depend essentially on the number and location of fibers that have been broken.

The first type of edged weapons are sharp pointed knives. They are called this because they act through a point, that when pressed in contact with skin separates the fibers and causes injury. Such 'stabbing' weapons can include a large number of tools such as chisels, awls, needles and so on. The only condition is that it has a sharp tip that breaks the skin.

Another very important factor is the thickness of the instrument, which is what controls the number of fibres they break. If the weapon, or instrument, is very thin, a needle for example, externally there is only going to be a red spot as a sign that there has been an injury.

If the instrument is thicker, like the ice-pick of Sharon Stone, there will be rupture of a larger number of fibers and the diameter of the hole will be greater. Another important element to consider in sharp instruments is their length, since this will affect the amount of harm done to internal organs.

So when there has been a sharp instrument wound, doctors should not trust the external appearance of the wound, as it may have reached the stomach, heart, a major artery, and so on. Therefore they should carry out exploratory investigations to rule out that it has injured some vital organ that has contributed to the death of the victim.

Another edged weapon that produces very characteristic injury is a knife with a single cutting edge. In this case the injury will be produced by a blade that has been pressed onto the skin or been used in a cutting motion.

Such instruments are kitchen knives, razor blades and scalpels, some other cutters, and some other tools that have a sharp edge. The wounds to which they may give rise to are varied, both in appearance and in severity. They range from simple cuts, of the type that we all get peeling a potato or opening a can of tuna, to even amputations.

Another important set of edged instruments are those formed of sharp pointed and edged cutting weapons, as you have probably guessed, with the characteristics of the two previous varieties. They have a point and also one, two or more sharp edges. Usually, having only one or two sharp edges, the most representative examples are hunting knives, daggers, letter openers, etc. The study of the wounds caused by sharp cutting instruments poses many challenges, but these are usually resolved by a comprehensive study of both the entry wound and the path it has followed inside the body.

Anyway, as I have said on other occasions, the study of these injuries cannot create a story of how things occurred, what can be done is to support or disprove a given hypothesis.

The last set of edged weapons are short, blunt instruments. They are those which have an edge, but they also have a substantial mass and are used with great force. The butchers' cleavers, axes and guillotines are three examples of such instruments. Usually they are weapons that cause very substantial injury, affecting both the skin and other soft tissues and bone structures. This was one of the reasons for developing the deadly instrument which proved to be so effective in France on countless occasions and whose invention was falsely attributed to Dr. Guillotin.

Having reviewed the edged weapons, used to injure since the dawn of time, let us see how human beings invented new gadgets to kill other humans.

Of course, another large group of instruments that can be used to injure and kill are guns. They are well known by the public, but we should say that, as in the case of edged weapons, they may be of many types. They may be long or short with one or two barrels, be automatic or semi-automatic and so on. They produce injuries from which, in many cases, we can draw a number of forensic inferences.

Actually the main information is obtained from the study of something that is common to all firearms. In all of them the projectile, or projectiles, are propelled towards the target, by the explosion of primer and powder in the cap or cartridge. Investigating all the effects that arise from this explosion enables the forensic scientists to draw many of their conclusions.

When the explosion occurs, as well as the projectile leaving the barrel there are the combustion gases that propel the projectile along with residues from the primer and unburnt grains of propellant. These are referred to as 'firearms discharge residues'. As each of these elements has a different effective range, detecting them, or not detecting them on skin or clothing of a person allows us to establish approximately the distance from which the shot has been fired.

Do you remember ever having heard the expression "shot him at point blank range"? That would mean that the weapon was at a distance from the body allowing the hot gases produced from the discharge to singe the clothes, or skin, of the victim. However, we must take into account two important aspects. The first is that when the distance is greater than the range of the firearm discharge residues it is impossible to establish from what distance the shot was made. The wounds of shots from great distances look similar to those from five, ten or twenty meters.

The second is that, for the proper interpretation of the facts where firearms are involved, if the shot has not hit bare skin one must examine the clothes worn by the victim at the time of being shot because they can act as a filter and retain firearm discharge residues. These may then assist in the interpretation and conclusions.

I could say a lot more about firearms, but if I dwell on them would be a pity because I could not then talk about another group of causes of death, frequent in medico-legal experience, which are those due to mechanical asphyxia. This term is used to describe a cause of death where there is a particular mechanism that impedes the victim's breathing. This includes hanging, strangulation, suffocation, blocking of the airway, thoracic-abdominal compression and lack of breathable air.

Drowning is also in this group by tradition, although the methods for establishing death differ significantly. Hanging is one of the best known forms of mechanical suffocation generally known by laymen. The image of a hanged man is familiar to everyone.

Remember that there is even a word guessing game that gets called this. I think it would be a much more acceptable, educational game, for example, if they drew a bed, instead of a scaffold, and the game would end when the puppet is wrapped up to go to bed, instead of when he it is hanged. It is just an idea.

For the forensic scientist the image of a hanged man can have very different aspects, given the number of possible ways of hanging. The mechanism that characterizes the hanging is a constriction of the neck where the weight of the body of the victim generates the force and death can be caused by four mechanisms.

The first is that the pressure of the noose prevents entry of air through the larynx; this would be a slow asphyxiation or choking to death.

The second is the noose prevents the normal circulation of blood to be maintained to the head, in which case the higher pressures occur laterally in the neck and normal flow to, or from, the head is prevented.

The latter may be called a blue hanging, if only the exiting of blood from the head is restricted and white if the pressure is higher and also prevents the flow of blood to the head. Death usually results more rapidly in the latter case than the former.

The third cause of death occurs because the hanging loop produces a stimulation of certain nerve endings in the neck region that make a virtually instantaneous cardiac arrest occur.

Finally, the fourth mechanism, the effect of the weight of the victim which can often fracture the bony structures of the neck and a section of the spinal column causing death instantaneously.

The importance of knowing exactly the cause of death is that, subsequently it will allow us to explain some other injuries that may have occurred to the body.

For example, a death by the first mechanism allows the body to have seizures and swing on the rope. If the body has bruises and scratches on some parts of the body they may have been produced by bumping against adjacent structures.

However, if the death was due to one of the instantaneous mechanisms, explanation of the other blows would not be so simple.

Death by strangulation is a mechanism that is immediately associated with the murder, but is not always necessarily the case. There are two basic types of strangulation: manual solely produced by use of the hands; and the use of a garrote.

In both cases there is a constriction of the neck, but unlike hanging, the force needed to compress that area is not generated by the weight of the individual, but by other mechanisms that may be caused by another person, or the victim, or by a mechanical agent.

The ways death occurs in strangulation are quite similar to those I have outlined for hanging, but it is virtually impossible for a broken neck to occur unless done deliberately or there is an enormous imbalance of strength between the victim and the assailant.

In gagging and suffocation and other mechanical asphyxia, things are quite clear and need little explanation. Blocking of the nostrils and mouth may occur with hands or with some other object.

In this regard there are in the medico-legal literature some cases where the breast of a careless mother feeding an infant claimed the life of the infant by smothering them.

Do not forget that in such cases, to cause death, the three breathing orifices that most of us have, must be blocked. The isolated occlusion of the nose or mouth does not have deadly consequences. If you do not believe me experiment and experience it yourselves; you doubting Thomases.

In occlusion of the airway the mechanism is asphyxia and as its name speaks for itself I feel no need for further clarification. Many of us have experienced the effects ourselves when we choked on some bread and wine.

Thoraco-abdominal compression is a mechanical asphyxia in which the impediment to respiration is established by applying a force on the ribs and abdomen, especially the upper part of it. This is less well-known than the previous one and it is possible to miss this mechanism which may be important.

Experiment; put the palms of your hands on the end of the ribs, with fingers extended pressing on the stomach and try to breathe deeply, it is difficult is it not? Well imagine if instead of the force you used, it is the weight of a man on the chest of a child or a marble slab on an adult.

Text books on forensic medicine report that this was the method used by the notorious murderers Burke and Hare in Edinburgh, Scotland, to kill homeless drunks and sell corpses for anatomical studies. The word 'burking' is sometimes used as a slang term in English for asphyxiation by compressing the chest of a victim.

The last type of asphyxia I will comment on is the lack of respirable, or breathable, air. This is exactly what the name indicates, in these cases death will always occur slowly, since breathable air does not usually suddenly disappear. A typical example of this type of death is that of a person who is locked in a room without any ventilation. Gradually, the oxygen is consumed and when there is no more, they die. Inevitably!

As in many other cases, when it is suspected that the death has been produced by a lack of respirable air, recording the time the corpse is recovered can provide valuable information on the cause of death.

Drowning asphyxiation is another mechanism that is traditionally studied in the group of mechanical asphyxia, although as I noted earlier, the causes of death are different.

It exceeds the scope of this book to make a comprehensive description of the problems posed by drowning and therefore I only point out a fact of great importance. When the medical examiner goes to sea the only sure thing is that he will be recovering a body from the water. Only when carrying the autopsy and using some additional techniques may he establish what the actual cause of death has been because the possibilities are many.

Let's see what they may be:

1. The individual has died of natural causes out of the water and has fallen into it after death.

2. They were in the water and died from natural causes, a heart attack perhaps, without further speculation.

3. They have been murdered out of the water and then been thrown into the sea.

4. They were enjoying themselves, in the water but died violently; either hit by a boat, or attacked by a wild, giant, killer crab.

5. They have died from the effects of ingesting seawater.

The preceding sentence also opens up several possibilities as follows:

6. It may be that the mere contact with the cold water will trigger the death and, therefore there is no intake of 'breath' under water, we would then have a case of *dry drowning.*

7. It may be that the subject because they are alive and unharmed immersed in water, cannot hold their breath any longer and attempts to 'breathe' underwater. The consequence is that the airways and lungs fill with water and these therefore are called *wet drownings.*

8. Finally, it is possible that the person receives a shock and losing consciousness, being immersed in water it enters into their lungs, killing them eventually.

Each of the possibilities I have mentioned leaves their particular indications on the body, hence the care with which we should carry out our examination, until we have exhausted all possibilities.

I consider, dear readers, that you already have a sufficient overview of some of the mechanisms of death investigated by a coroner. I have mentioned some of the ones which occur most frequently in practice in more detail but, of course, there are many other possibilities; the effects of electricity, be it natural or artificial, the effects of heat and cold, radiation, explosions, burns from fire or chemical agents, etc.., are a few of them.

Probably elsewhere in this booklet I will make reference to some of them, but it will be from a different point of view than I have tried to use in this chapter.

I would point out finally, that although I have spoken of intentional poisoning, the study of poisons and their effects on the body would justify a very extensive chapter on its own.

Come on. We will not keep him in suspense. The coroner is waiting to see if the pathologist can tell us more.

CHAPTER

7

Was it murder, suicide or an accident?

This is undoubtedly a crucial question for many people; especially for friends and relations of the deceased. However, while each of these possibilities has very different consequences; for forensic medicine it is just another problem to solve.

In this chapter I will discuss some of the effects that are studied in cadavers and the physical and social environments in which they have been found. In scientific terms this is known as the forensic etiology of the death.

Addressing this problem properly is a substantial programme of work. We are trying to differentiate between natural and violent, or unnatural, deaths. This is the first question that must be answered in the investigation of a death, since, on this, subsequent actions and possible judicial intervention and accountabilities depend.

Deaths are referred to as natural if there are no external agents or causes to initiate them. They include all deaths caused by any disease process that we can imagine: myocardial infarction, spontaneous cerebral hemorrhage, respiratory failure, kidney or liver disease, intestinal obstruction, leukemia, etc.

Those caused by infections are also usually natural deaths even though, in most cases, the micro-organisms responsible come from outside the body. We say these are 'innocent agents' which cannot be blamed for having caused the death. Remember however, what I said about the mechanisms of direct and indirect death. If any of the conditions I have outlined above, is triggered by an external event, whether active or passive, we find ourselves dealing with the kinds of death described below.

As opposed to natural deaths, we meet violent, or unnatural, deaths, which are due to the action of multiple and various external agents. In this group there are three possible types of actions of the external agent that ultimately give rise to three possible conclusions: homicide, suicide and accident. In the case of homicides, one or more people, more or less intentionally, are responsible for the events that initiate the cause of death.

There are times that the intention is not to kill, but it results in a death nevertheless. At other times, the object of the action is, indeed, to cause the death of another person.

From these and other factors, some of them obviously medico-legal, arise the potential criminal charges that a judicial system may initiate as a result of the death. These are murder, manslaughter, dangerous driving, assault with intent to cause grievous bodily harm, etc. In suicides, or self-inflicted deaths, there is an external mechanism, but the characteristic is that it is the victim that sets it in motion.

Nor in these cases is it possible to talk about only one type of suicide. So, in many cases the cause of death is deliberately triggered and there has been enough planning for it to succeed. In other cases however, there are attempted suicides, or 'parasuicides', which actually aim to draw the attention of people close to the victim. Unfortunately sometimes things just do not go according to plan and the suicide attempt results in death.

Finally, another large group are spontaneous self-inflicted deaths, suicides actually, but characterized by a sudden decision to end their own life. In these cases there is not the premeditation and planning shown in the first type. The fundamental issue when it is established that a death is suicide, is that there is no need to look for another person to attribute it to. Only in cases where there is intervention, or assistance, of another person should further investigation be carried out.

In accidental deaths, unlike the previous cases, there is no human intent that has set in motion the mechanism by which death has occurred. I will emphasise this, because it is a key point: although another person may be involved in producing an accident, the important thing is that such involvement is unintentional.

For example, in certain industrial accident cases death may result from the non-compliance of a third party with safety regulations. But the death will not have been caused by the direct or expressed intention of another.

As you will have come to realize in this chapter, causes of death can be very different and also they may kill some time after the critical event occurred. That is why, in all cases where there was an accident or an incident of some consequence, and although time has elapsed since the event, there should be an autopsy to establish a possible relationship between the events and the subsequent death.

If there is another person implicated, they may be made to accept appropriate responsibilities. Accidental deaths are not so often encountered in forensic medicine.

There are also cases in which, whilst not being a natural death, it is not possible to find a responsible person. A typical case of this type of violent death is someone killed by being struck by lightning. Unless we are going to search for someone dressed in white with a long beard, or someone in red with horns, these are usually regarded as 'Acts of God'.

I should say from a number of reports that this type of incident can usually be regarded as an 'accident'.

The investigation of industrial accidents may involve a number of very specialist circumstances and technicalities beyond the scope of this volume.

Turning now to the forensic science issues, the first thought by investigators when approaching the diagnosis of accidental death, suicide or homicide should be to consider the environment, the social and physical surroundings, of the victim. Of course it is not the job of the medical examiner to investigate these. This is the duty of the judicial and prosecuting authorities adjudicating on the death.

It is time to find reasons and the cause of death. "Cherchez la femme", the French say. In suicide and homicide there is a huge range of possible causes which could explain why they happen. In some cases the causes may be remote, while in others there is a clear series of events in which the last link is the death.

Cases of suicide have been linked, among others, to such factors as: mental illness, emotional distress, job loss, educational failure, financial problems, the exposure of an economic or political scandal, the fear of the end of the world, neglect by relatives - in the case of the elderly, contracting an incurable illness, death of a close family member, etc.

The relegation of a football team to a lower league has claimed more than one victim by suicide.

I have listed above situations which occur to very many people, but fortunately these do not result in a similar number of suicides. This is because it also requires a certain personality, or a bias toward self-destruction, and limited capacity to cope with such setbacks.

If there are more than one of the above triggering factors the probability that suicide has occurred is correspondingly increased. In murder usually the same happens; there is always something to explain why it was carried out.

Actually I would say that, in my opinion, there is never any reason to kill someone.

It is difficult to understand why we still frequently see newspapers headlines such as: "He killed his brother for no reason".

As in the other type of violent death, in homicides we also find a wide range of circumstances; some very diverse stories involving, drugs, prostitution, criminal activities, terrorism, robbery, sexual assault, family disagreements. A high proportion of cases of homicides everywhere result from family feuds, love rivalries, disputes in drinking bars, rivalries among urban gangs, clashes over land boundaries or irrigation, 'road rage', political rivalries and very many 'etceteras' for other motives.

Along with all these we need to consider two special cases.

The first is that of someone who is mentally disturbed and who is responsible for the death of a person as a direct consequence of their mental state. In these events, the medical examiner must also consider the assailant's illness and relate it to what he has done.

The broad field of Forensic Psychiatry, as with the study of poisons and poisoning, also deserves an entire book.

The other special case is one in which death occurs 'just because' for no real reason. Killing for killing's sake; coldly and without any real reason.

One example is the deaths that have occurred as part of so-called 'role playing groups'. It is difficult to investigate the facts, but particularly difficult because there may be nothing on the body, or at the scene, to implicate the perpetrator or perpetrators.

Precisely because of this, I must stress the extreme importance of the three phases of examination: the state of the body when removed from the scene, the investigation of the crime scene itself and the external review of the body; primarily in the clothes worn and then unclothed.

During those three stages we must be especially meticulous, given that, very probably, what we do not find then, and note, photograph or video, in those initial phases, will be difficult to establish later. Do not ignore anything, since later it may prove to be crucial.

WHAT ABOUT SOME EXAMPLES?

The discovery of a lit gas stove where a body is found.

The way some blood stains have been cleaned up on a floor or wall.

Cigarette butts in an ashtray, or collected off the floor.

The height of a stool found in a place where there was a hanging.

Tickets or currency found in clothes on a skeleton.

The way the hands of a body were tied.

Half-eaten chewing gum or candy.

Here is, of course, another possible long list of 'etceteras' of items and details that can provide information that then may become relevant evidence. Yes, it may be a waste of time, but we will only know that when it has been gathered and investigated.

I have already covered several specific types of death which may be accident, suicide or homicide. I will try to highlight those aspects that can assist physicians in establishing the final diagnosis, but with the caveat that the final decision is that of the magistrate or coroner when all lines of enquiry which have been opened are completed.

SHOOTINGS

The study of the wounds caused by firearms, to establish the forensic etiology of their production, is based on a number of procedures and methods, some of which are apparently easy to interpret, but which actually must be very carefully evaluated.

As I noted in another chapter, there are many types of firearms. In the following paragraphs I will consider a case study involving a short barreled non-automatic pistol.

A body of a man is found in a room of his home, he is shot in the right temple and there is a gun in his hand, and he is indeed dead. Other circumstances may be gradually be uncovered.

On one hand, the police are investigating the circumstances and surroundings of the man's life, seeking to establish whether anything in the life of the deceased person could lead to some clues as to reasons for his death. On the other hand, forensic scientists will be looking for where the bullet is, either at the scene or at the autopsy, and finding out whether it came from the same gun as found at the scene.

Medical examiners will check whether the shot was made at a distance compatible with the length of the arm of the victim. Also considering the direction in which the shot was fired and whether that is commensurate with this distance. Also determining whether there are traces of firearms discharge residues on the hands, depending on the distance and direction the gun has been held at. Usually the determined suicide uses both hands.

They must also check that the death was due to the gunshot wound and no other different earlier mechanism, such as food poisoning or other head injury. They will also be determining whether the shot was the fatal wound, with the techniques I reflected on in another chapter.

The presence of drugs in the blood must be investigated, since, for example, a high level of tranquilizers, can deprive a person of understanding of the act of suicide. But it could also have been in preparation to commit murder.

After each specialist, criminal, forensic or medical, has completed their examination the information is collated and presented to the prosecutors or coroner to determine what further proceedings will be initiated.

Naturally, the process of investigating a case, that I have tried to summarize briefly, is very complex. It is therefore not surprising that proceedings subsequent to the death of a person in a case of suicide, homicide or accident, can take a very long time.

Cases of suicide with a firearm may occur in apparently very suspicious circumstances. The personality of the suicide can result, not infrequently, in self-destruction in strange and unusual ways.

An example is the body of a young man with a wound, gun shot in the back of the head; to make it clearer, at a point diametrically opposite the tip of the chin. One meter behind the body is a rifle and it is subsequently found that this is the weapon responsible. It appears that this is a murder, with the characteristics of an 'execution'. Following the completion of the investigation it was concluded that it was an atypical suicide. The person had taken the rifle with both hands, behind his back, looked upwards then with the gun barrel to the back of the head and fired.

As you can see, you can't tell a book by its cover.

DEATHS AND ARSON.

It is well known that setting fire to a house or a vehicle is a frequently used method for trying to conceal the commission of crime. I pointed this out to a friend and faculty colleague, we have also seen this done in many films. In these cases it is essential to exhaust all the possibilities offered by forensic medicine, not taking anything for granted.

In a building where there has been a fire many possible causes of death may be found and each one of them is going to leave a series of signs that, if properly studied will enable valuable conclusions to be reached.

Death may be due to the direct effect of flames, by the effects of carbon monoxide, the gas generated by incomplete combustion of various flammable materials, by injuries from the collapsing building, by poisoning with other gases produced by the combustion of plastics, or by jumping from the building.

If the fire was caused by an explosion, or an electrical fault, death may also have resulted from this initiation mechanism. However, it is very suspicious when a body found after a fire, is shown to have died due to a gunshot, a stab wound, hanging or strangulation. It is strange, but of course it has happened.

As I said before, each of the causes of death that I have referred to leaves signs and their location and interpretation is the job of the forensic scientists. For example, in the case of finding a body in the burned remains of a factory, one of the first things you have to do is find out if the deceased has breathed, a little or a lot, while the fire was burning.

This is done by examining the airways, the trachea and bronchi, as where breathing has occurred these areas will have traces from the combustion process in the form of soot particles or other traces of smoke from the environment. If they also have a skull fracture, by application of appropriate techniques, we will be able to determine if those injuries occurred before or after death.

These are only some of the types of information and observations that medical examiners, or pathologists, contribute to an investigation.

But of course the inquest may clarify:

i. That the deceased is the owner of the factory.

ii. Who he has named sole heir to property.

iii. That the owner's wife is the mistress of the manager.

iv. That at the last audit an embezzlement of 30,000 dollars was detected

v.   That the manager is a pyromaniac ....

STABBING WOUNDS

With these types of weapons we should consider a number of issues when trying to establish if it is a homicide, suicide or an accident.

The body of a butcher is found where the meat is cut in his shop. He has a long and deep cutting wound on the left anterior side of the neck. In his right hand there is a knife. Underneath the body is a partly de-boned ham.

Questions:

Has he had an accident, by his own hand, while working?

Has he decided to end his life, ruined by the disastrous state of his business?

Has he been surprised by someone who had a score to settle with him?

I must make another point: at the introduction of this small volume I pointed out that the term forensic medical examiner, or pathologist, refers to a person with a specific responsibility in law. Well this is a case in which, theoretically at least, we will need the intervention of another forensic expert. We need a 'forensic butcher' who could tell the coroner the usual way to de-bone a ham. This would provide additional information to decide if it could indeed have been an accident.

Do we continue with the enigma of the dead butcher? Okay, but do not expect extravagant descriptions……only some basic information.

Ah! I forgot to say that the butcher was left handed. If it was an accident while working, we should see various aspects in agreement.

For example, the direction of the cut should be compatible with the movements necessary for cutting the meat from the bone. Usually this will be a clean cut, from front to back and with a fairly uniform depth.

The hand that wields the knife must be stained with blood, but in a manner consistent with the type of injury. The other hand must also be stained with blood, as a result of trying to stop the bleeding.

That it was a suicide should be doubted, since a left-handed person will usually cut into the right side of neck and right-hander on the left hand side. They are usually cut from back to front and often accompanied by other less deep cuts, which are attempts. Depth_of cut is usually also variable, deeper at the start and less deep at the end of the cut. Hands and clothing should also be stained, but, remember, in a manner consistent with the type of injury.

If it had been a homicide, it is also rather unusual, as in cutting a throat, murderers usually cut the front of the neck. In this case, the depth would also be variable, but in a manner contrary to suicide: less deep at the beginning and more in the last section of the wound, as if to ensure the result.

The direction could be as before, or reversed, depending on whether the murderer is right or left-handed. Staining of hands and clothing should be found in a way consistent with the mode of attack.

Do not be misled. I have given above just three simple examples. There are many more things to be studied, and then, later, they may be compared with the various hypotheses resulting from the judicial inquiry. We should never forget that there are extremely rare possibilities that nevertheless sometimes actually happen.

DEATH BY HANGING OR STRANGULATION

If you consider that to get rid of someone you can pretend that they have hanged themselves, don't even think of it! You cannot get away with it. Either with the decision to kill someone, or the method chosen. It may seem simple to kill a person then hang them from a rope. I believe that now you will be well prepared and not make simple mistakes;   but there can never be sufficient preparation and it is so obvious that we cannot misinterpret what has happened.

Hopefully they will not think that they can kill the poor victim with six gun shots and stab wounds in the back, and then hang them. That would be simple matter for the Court

It would be logical.... let me think ... ... to give them a potion or poison or ... give a blow to the head ... to cover their mouth and nose with a pillow ... or strangle them ... or submit them to a continuous session of jokes... and then hang the body.

Really, do not try because the chances of it going wrong are very high.

Apparently strangulation could be a possibility, but in reality, it is virtually impossible to achieve. Recalling the details in hanging deaths the different methods leave their mark on the body. Each of these mechanisms is related, amongst other things, to the position in which we find the noose around the neck, the weight of the body and the place where it has been hanging, and so on.

The situation, continuity, depth and texture of the grooves left on the neck, in hanging and strangulation are radically different. Therefore, the likelihood of a botched 'cover up' is enormous. Even if you put the rope around the neck of the victim as if he hanged himself you will find that it will still be spotted by the medical examiner.

The lesions that occur in the neck at the time of killing would have a vital characteristic reaction, referred to in another chapter. However, when the body is suspended on the rope, to simulate the hanging, there would be other injuries, this time on a corpse, they would not have any of the important characteristics.

DEATH AND DRUGS

Cases of deaths from drug administered intravenously, still occur frequently and are always disturbing, and always raise doubts about the forensic etiology. The most common occurrence is when the body of a person is found in some lonely place with the needle stuck in the arm near the flexure of the elbow. It is possible that the death occurred accidentally, but it could also fit the other two possibilities; suicide and homicide.

When it comes to accidental deaths, and where the person administering the drug did not intend to cause the death, there may be various explanations.

One is that the addict is accustomed to a given dose of drug, but has been without any for a while, either having been in jail, or has been trying to give up drugs, or has not been able to get the drugs on the streets, etc.

For whatever reasons, the fact is that when they resume use of the drug, the body is no longer able to support the dose as before and if they inject the same amount to which they were used, it can be a reaction to this that results in their death.

Another possibility relates to the drug suppliers. In these cases there may be, among others, two basic mechanisms.

The first is that, because drugs are in short supply, or to seek higher returns, they 'cut' the drug with a toxic substance, strychnine, is one that is used quite frequently, which brutality! Death may then be due to the action of the adulterant and not the principle drug. Other times, even when drugs are in short supply, the 'cut' products may not be unduly toxic and do not cause such serious harm to users.

Problems can also arise when there is easier availability of heroin and the proportion of the drug is higher, if the addict's body has become accustomed to a lower dose of heroin, the chance of having an adverse reaction are very high. Suicide in these cases cannot however necessarily be excluded, since in many cases, addicts live in very unpleasant circumstances and it is no surprise that sometimes they self-administer a dose they know they will not be able to tolerate.

Finally, homicide by drugs by the methods I have already outlined earlier. Simply replacing the usual supply by one with either very high heroine content or an adulterant as deadly as strychnine. The effects are distressing.

I will finish here; I could continue giving examples of other ways to die in which questions may arise about the origin of the actual triggering mechanism, but it could be rather like garlic, repeating on us. Being hit by vehicles, drownings, electrocutions, deaths on the railway, falls and the almost endless ways to die violently each having different indications depending on their nature. As I indicated at the beginning of the chapter, a thorough examination by the medical examiner along with the judicial investigation will clarify the situation in a great majority of cases.

There are times however, when someone dies, the body is buried, time passes and then the question ....

"Medical examiner can you tell us more?"

Close the book, drink some water, turn off the of the bedside light and sleep... or not.

That is the chapter for tomorrow.

CHAPTER

8

Will it help to exhume the body?

Sometimes, for more or less sensational reasons, there appears an announcement in the newspapers that a body is to be exhumed to determine some aspects of the cause of death which may not have been clear at the time of interments.

Sometimes there is news of the discovery of human remains somewhere and people expect that carrying out an autopsy will reveal the full facts of the case. In particular of course the main interest is the identity of the deceased and the circumstances surrounding their death.

These events take on a dramatic turn when presented in conjunction with lists of missing people. We will see in this chapter what forensic medicine can achieve in these cases.

To start on a cheerful, optimistic and relaxed note, I think it is worth making a reference to our local Regulations for Police Mortuary Health, which is state-wide Valencian legislation that controls many aspects, related to cadavers, that I mentioned in a previous chapter. Obviously I will not go on at length, but merely select those points which are more closely related to the issue to address in this penultimate section of the book.

The policy states that the possible final destinations of a corpse are in a mausoleum or burial ground, burial at sea, or cremation. It also indicates the time limits that cannot be exceeded without burying a body or conducting some preservation procedures.

Elsewhere in the book, I have already mentioned that you cannot carry out the burial of a body within 24 hours of the death of the person.

In the event that the burial is to occur between 48 hours and 72 hours after death, to avoid health risk certain basic preservation procedures should be carried out. These involve the application of a number of liquid and solid agents that delay decay of the cadaver but do not stop it completely. Lastly, when the burial of the body is to take place more than 72 hours after death, embalming must be undertaken, which, if done properly, prevents putrefaction of the corpse.

As you will already have sharply perceived, in cases where the embalming procedures have been carried out, the possibility that the forensic examiners can extract information of value on exhumation is considerably increased.

There is something else that is obvious. When the body has been cremated there is little you can do. But we can still try. We will look at that later.

In the chapter that I dedicated to determining the time of the death I gave some brief information on the decay of a corpse. I will now resume the description of this phenomenon, but from a different perspective. I intend to show how, although the body is in an 'advanced state of decomposition', words that are systematically repeated in the media, you may still find out many things.

There are no differences in techniques or methods to answer our questions.

In the first phase of the putrefactive process, known as chromatic or colored, the signs can be observed in a fresh corpse. In the second stage of putrefaction, the breakdown of body tissue and production of gases there are some effects that can lead to confusion, especially to non-experts.

The identification of the body may be somewhat more difficult because as well as the changes in the skin colors of the previous phase there is the bloating of the body. The gases accumulated inside the body cause the chest, abdomen and the face, primarily due to changes in the eyes and tongue, to deform dramatically.

I remember now that the following headline appeared a newspaper in Valencia: 'It appears that a black man has been murdered in a plot'.

After two or three days, and after the autopsy had been conducted, the newspaper could not find a better way to correct this than say: "The black man who was found murdered in the plot was white."

In cases where there is extensive swelling of the body, we must be especially careful with the interpretation of two possible aspects.

One is that death sometimes comes to someone wearing a shirt and tie, if in this situation, putrefaction progresses there will be a time when the accumulated gas has distended the neck. Then the clothes they wore become tight around the neck and can leave a mark looking like a ligature or strangulation. So, be careful!

Another is that, with advancing putrefaction spontaneous skin ruptures due to, on the one hand, the degeneration of tissues, and on the other the build up of gas pressure.

So when we see these areas of damage, apparently wounds, we must differentiate whether they are due to the bloating or, conversely, that they are actual wounds for example inflicted by a weapon.

The putrefaction is continuously advances, like any midfield footballer worth his salt, and reaches the third stage or liquefaction phase.

Here things get more complicated because during the liquefaction stage the various tissues lose their shape and tend to form masses so that it is difficult to recognize things. The various organs undergo this degradation at different speeds depending on their nature.

For example, heart and uterus will degrade slower than the liver and lungs. Therefore, if it is suspected that a death resulted from an injury to the heart, it is easier to detect than if the death may have been produced after haemorrhage from a ruptured liver.

The fact that the uterus as an organ is quite resistant to putrefaction has considerable value as when a corpse is found, even in a very advanced state of putrefaction, it is possible to reliably establish the sex.

You know, in another chapter, that the end of the liquefaction stage of putrefaction is the formation of a sort of mass referred to in Spanish as *pastosilla* or *putrílago*. Note that even the name inspires some aversion.

The last stage of putrefaction is called the skeletal reduction phase. The *putrílago* disappears and there are only, nails, hair and bones connected by ligaments. Finally, over many, many years, everything other than the bones disappears too. When only bones are exhumed from a grave there is still the possibility of some forensic evidence being obtained.

In such cases, of course, complete skeletons are much more valuable than isolated bones although even then investigation should not be abandoned.

In fact, one of the first tasks that must be tackled when bones arrive at a forensic anthropology laboratory is to establish the number of subjects from which the various skeletal elements belong. The investigation is of course constrained by something very important, it has to be established at the lab that they are human bones.

This diagnosis of species is usually resolved very easily when you have complete skeletons. Things become more difficult when there are only bone fragments. In such cases usually immunoanalysis techniques enable us to discard those not of human origin.

Regarding identification, there are many things to do. We can establish the sex of the corpse from the skeleton drawing on the fact that there are substantial differences between men and women. Among others, the configuration of parts of the skull, the shape of the pelvis, the areas where tendons attach to bones, the thickness of the bones, and so on.

The race, height and age are other identifying features that we may try to establish with anthropological techniques.

Getting closer to determining the racial type of the remains can be achieved by studying the morphological characteristics of the skull or jaw and by other methods, such as establishing the relationships between the size of the skull and other bones of the body. We can also investigate the relationships between length, width and curvature of various components of the skeleton.

Regarding age, the first thing to note is that the techniques used will vary depending on how old approximately we think, the person, the 'owner' of the bones, may have been. Thus, we will not employ exactly the same techniques when, apparently, the remains belong to a small child, as when it is likely to be an old man.

Even with this caveat, the methods are very similar, as we use the knowledge we have about the rate of the processes of ossification of the people, from birth to old age.

The study of points of ossification of various bones, fusion of their zones of elongation, which occur when the individual has stopped growing, and the study of cranial suture closure, among others, are the methods that offer greatest reliability.

Please excuse me if I make a clarification: the diagnosis of sex is always more accurate than of the age;

due, among other things to the fact that one can only be male or female.

In the case of age, medico-legal reports are not precise; the results are presented in the form of an age range (10 to 14 years, over 65 years, etc.).

As for height, when you have the complete skeleton, we add together the measurements of the various components, and then making a correction to compensate for the absence of soft or semi-soft tissues, which also contributes to our height. When only isolated bones are available, we can calculate a relationship between the length of them and the subject's overall stature, but this will only give an approximation.

There are some reports by authors who have established relationships between the lengths of the teeth and the height of the body to which they belong.

Continuing with identification, the fact that the person whose body we are studying has suffered some type of bone disease or an accident with fractures, is of great importance. These changes leave permanent signs in the bones that are readily apparent.

In addition there remains dental identification, facial reconstruction by computer or by clay reconstruction and the study of the DNA.

And, even if we find an identity card on the skeleton, apparently making identity clear; this should not be used as a reason not to carry out the identification procedures. Appearances, you know, are deceptive.

Some possible causes of death may also be investigated on skeletal remains but obviously, only in certain cases and with considerable caution   As an illustrative example, in the depths of a lush forest, a skeleton is found and beside it a rifle.

The pathologist noted that the skull has a hole and initially deemed that it is compatible with being produced by a firearm.

After conducting all the necessary studies, and confirming that indeed this is a hole caused by a projectile, you still need to consider whether some characteristic features have been produced in life or after death.

If it were possible to establish in this exceptional case that the individual was alive when he was shot what could the coroner say about what happened.

I make a suggestion: shut the book and try to develop possible scenarios that may have occurred.

Overcome the temptation and do not continue reading, because in the following paragraphs there are some solutions. Please!

Thank you for the effort.

Let's see the answers. We might propose that, theoretically:

1. The man was walking in the country and an individual (passing by) shot him in the head.

2 . The man was tired of life and decided to shoot himself in the head.

3. The man was hunting, tripped over, fell to the ground and accidentally fired a shot that struck him in the head and killed him.

4. The man suffered a major brain hemorrhage that killed him and in the fall to the ground, the gun accidentally discharged, hitting him in the head.

If you have come up with broadly the same four theories proposed by the coroner, there are valuable prizes.

I suggest you go and treat yourself to a ticket for the National Lottery!

Of course I have to admit that the only certainty may be that the cause of death was a gunshot to the head. All I tried to clarify with the exercise was to show that very often the investigators cannot come to categorical conclusions.

One last thing about skeletons. When death may have been due to poisoning there are times when we can get information from the bones. There are some poisons that are stored in the bone structure and therefore even over time the possibility of detection remains.

In such cases we must be careful since contamination can occur from the surroundings where the remains have been found and lead to false interpretations and conclusions.

At the beginning of this chapter I pointed out the possibility that a body may have been treated or embalmed to delay the phenomena of putrefaction and that this could facilitate the forensic investigations of the coroner as some evidential signs could remain for longer.

Well, the same phenomenon of conservation of the corpse can occur naturally and may be by a so called saponification or by mummification processes.

The medico-legal value of each is different, because in most cases, the saponified bodies eventually decompose similar to normal cadavers, but mummification may cause bodies to last for tens or even hundreds of years.

Let's see what these processes are.

Saponification is a process in which various body tissues are transformed into types of derived fats which quite accurately depict the external shape of the body.

The internal organs are not transformed and usually suffer the normal process of putrefaction.

For this natural preservation to occur you have to have certain environmental conditions; very high humidity, lack of ventilation, and a certain obese constitution, or some disease or illness which in the living causes the degeneration of fatty tissue.

When this occurs it forms a kind of fatty mantle which starts as oily skin and deepens into the other tissue.

Being a process of substitution, we will meet with some limitations.

For example, fingerprints are not retained, as the original skin has been replaced by fat tissue which does not have the fineness of detail needed to provide the ridge detail.

If there has been an injury to the skin it will not be preserved, since it changes to fat, all that could be perceived is a certain difference in the texture and color of the fat occupying the area where the wound was.

Finally, as I have already mentioned, the internal organs are not preserved so it will be impossible to establish a link between external marks and internal injuries that may have caused death.

Mummification, as discussed below, is a far more useful phenomenon. To avoid confusion I should point out that when we speak of 'mummies' in forensic terms, we are not referring to those that you are familiar with their bandages, their arms folded across their chest, in a sarcophagus in their pyramid, and so on. They are 'artificial' mummies.

Natural mummification is a process in which there is a rapid drying of the tissue. Lacking water, the bacteria that were due to initiate putrefaction can not develop and die. It follows logically, in the sense that a person is like a bacterium, they may both die of thirst.

To form a mummy there are also a number of necessary environmental conditions, low humidity, free flowing ventilation, high temperature, constitutional requirements, slim, or pathological conditions, death from dehydration or bleeding. When these circumstances occur, skin and other tissues dry quickly and there is insufficient time for the bacteria of putrefaction to start their work.

With regard to the identification of a mummified corpse I note two relevant points.

The first is that the skin is not replaced by anything, but has simply dried. Therefore, obtaining fingerprints information is possible after applying a tissue regenerative procedure.

The second, less common, is that tattoos, which are an identifier of considerable value, will remain perfectly recognizable as the mummy does not deteriorate with the passage of time.

Regarding the possible determination of the cause of death, remember that the skin of a shriveled mummy looks; I insist that they have nothing to do with the Egyptians; the same for a long time, including any wounds and other signs of trauma.

If we add that the internal organs may have also been mummified, it is then possible to establish a relationship between a 'wound' in front of the chest of the mummy and an injury for example to the heart.

To round off the chapter, I will clarify what I meant when referring to the cases of cremations.

I said that, even in these cases, the medical examiner may be able to extract some useful information.

If the death of an individual is produced by the action of a knife, or any other such injury mechanism, the incineration process will wipe out any trace that could clarify the matter.

However, if you might suspect the death to have been caused by poison it would not be unreasonable to try to get some data. The first necessary condition for this is that the poison used is one that resists the effects of the high temperatures generated in the crematoria.

The second condition is very basic: the urn containing the ashes must be located, either in the home or in one of the repositories that exist in the cemeteries, especially dedicated to the disposal of ashes.

If these two conditions are met then a toxicological analysis must be carried out to reveal the existence of abnormally large amounts of the poison being investigated.

The presence of the poison would be the objective fact: there is much poison XXX for example. However, always wise, the pathologist must investigate other aspects.

Among other things, whether the materials used to build the coffin or the paint also contains poison XXX or if anything else may have been put in the coffin beside the body that might contain it.

As you have come to realize, the passage of time can blur boundaries and hinder medico-legal interpretation of some data. But in every case the practitioners of Forensic Medicine should try to offer their best assistance to the administration of justice.

We are nearing the end and, as in any medico-legal report there remains the conclusions.

CHAPTER
9

Conclusions

Finishing work is always difficult especially written work. Because even if you look at it and check again and again, one can always find things missing or out of place. In fact, if I continue reviewing the chapters, I run the real risk of having to change the title to "What the great-great-grandfather of the pathologist said?"

In the introduction and the seven thematic chapters I have collected examples of some of the many types of investigation that medical examiners or pathologists undertake in the course of our work.

My intention has been for you to understand how much we can do and what limitations and restrictions there are that can affect what we can interpret from observations of a corpse. Only you can say if this has been worthwhile, I have used personal experiences and forensic medical knowledge that has been accumulated over the history of our science.

We must not forget that the progress of science is always the result of the contributions of great creative minds and meticulous observers, together with many other anonymous individuals who have contributed their grains of sand. All of which has the central objective of improving accuracy and understanding.

Nevertheless, although the purpose of the scientific progress is generally to benefit humanity – this is still limited by ignorance and prejudice. Any discovery must wait for those not so well versed in the art, to become enlightened and to join in.

An example of this is found in the vicissitudes suffered over the years in the investigation of paternity. Blood tests for paternity testing, with an accuracy very close to one hundred percent were known 'medically' long before they were accepted by the legal authorities in many countries. In Spain, this recognition came with the enactment of the current Constitution in 1978. The acceptance of a breakthrough is limited by the attitudes of mind which vary with different cultures and times. Ideas too advanced for one age may be accepted, without reservation, fifty or a hundred years later; ask Leonardo da Vinci, and let us not forget Leonardo's ideas had a sound scientific basis. They were not merely wild speculations conflicting with established scientific knowledge.

Forensic Medicine is not a new science; not at all; if you do not believe me carry on reading; from its early development it has been inextricably linked to the evolution and history of medicine from its earliest times.

As a start I want to mention something not often considere, the first being who performed a forensic medicine investigation was the hominid that, based on their observations, was able to generalise about what they saw in their fellow beings. I think we can agree that, without doubt, in those remote times, they would be able to diagnose death.

The documented history of science is currently believed to begin with the Code of Ur-Namnu (2,500 BC), and later the Code of Hammurabi in 1700 BC; in this there are several references to problems in which forensic medicine was relevant, in medical liability cases, rape, abortions, etc.

The Law of Moses in its various texts focuses on issues that are also considered closely related to Forensic Medicine. Thus one finds references to menstruation, marriage, abortion, pregnancy and childbirth, standards for burials, etc. In this Law special attention is paid to the obligation to compensate for injuries that have been inflicted on a person during an assault. Criteria are used to try to balance the compensation with the amount of injury caused; well-known as 'an eye for an eye'. It could not be otherwise, today something similar to this is in the Spanish Penal Code where crimes against the individual are considered.

It is generally accepted that the greatest contributions to legal medicine, by ancient cultures, have come from China. Many people may think it is much more recent, but in third century China physicians could be specifically trained to intervene to resolve legal disputes. Between 138BC and 201BC someone known as Galen, made many contributions to our field of science. These included a treaty on feigned diseases and, most importantly, the so called hydrostatic pulmonary docimasia, a technique that even today is used to resolve some cases of infant death.

It is well known that early examples of the codification of laws are documented in the history of Rome; this includes brief references to some laws having medical or biological associations. In the Roman Law of the Twelve Tables, *Leges XII tabularum,* there are various biological and medical provisions recorded. As examples the law on 'an eye for an eye' was modified, and reference made to possibility of establishing paternity by the period of gestation.

Julius Caesar was murdered forty-four years before the birth of Jesus Christ. You must remember the scene from a movie where a large number of senators, stabbed the Emperor. It was a physician, Antistius, who established that, of the wounds received, only one in the thorax was a fatal wound. Even today this question is frequently asked of medical examiners before the courts. Which of all the wounds present in a body has caused the death? Of course it is easy to understand that the consequences for the assailants can be very different depending on the answer given.

In the fifth century Germanic and Slav barbarian tribes standardized *wéhgeld* penalties for injury compensation using medical experts. If you had injured someone, you had to pay him, or his family, as awarded by the Court *weh* = damage or harm, *geld* = money. The historical significance of this is that the Court took the advice of a medical expert. Now this type of medical expertise is referred to as Personal Injury Assessment, which is a part of Legal Medicine of considerable social and economic significance.

The *Salic Law* (485-511) establishes the compulsory involvement of a 'competent person' to examine the wounded and issue the advice before setting compensation.

The *Koran,* contains various aspects of legislation and some of its verses speak of adoption, homicide, menstruation, wills, incest, adultery, the law of retribution and so on.

The power of the papacy in Italy in the thirteenth century is noted by historians as a landmark for the establishment of a medical intervention in certain court cases.

Pope Innocent II, 1209AD, and then the Pope Gregory IX, 1257AD, instituted medical intervention as a necessary legal requirement for the better administration of justice. In epistles by the latter there were references to laws relating to various issues with significant medical or biological content: marriage, disability, fatal injuries, impotence, cesareans, abortions, etc.

In Spain during the Middle Ages there was a period of transition from traditional rules and customs and the establishment of a statutory legal body, framework and hierarchy. It started with the Fuero Juzgo a codex of Spanish laws which spread out from Castile to other areas setting out rules and giving the population certain rights and privileges. The administration in Old Castile was the first to set a scale of penalties for compensation for assaults causing injuries. This is very relevant, because the great majority of compensation claims in our courts are dealt with based on standardized scales.

Alfonso X, El Sabio (The Wise One), introduced in 1255 some rules for use of the courts. At the same time he commanded the compilation of laws, known as the Royal Charter for general adoption. His legislative efforts culminated with the writing of Las Siete Partidas which discusses various aspects of law.

An unusual aspect of this compilation was that each book began with a letter of the name of the King:

Book I **(A).** Natural and ecclesiastical law.

Book II **(L)** Political Law.

Books III to VI **(F, O, N, S)** civil and private sectors.

Finally, Book VII **(O)** Penal Code.

The main medico-legal aspects in this work are: the authorization for medical practice and intervention; the criminal responsibility of the mentally ill and their business capacity; marriage and some of its problems.

The practice of dissection of human cadavers was not yet widespread in Spain during this period. However, after the introduction of this in the Faculty of Medicine of Montpellier in 1340, you can see how, in turn, provided by royal authority, it was established in several

Spanish cities: Lerida in 1391, Barcelona in 1401, Valencia in 1477 and Zaragoza in 1488.

To outline the most important facts of the so-called modern period in the development of the Legal Medicine I will relate them to the perspective of the major social movements.

THE RENAISSANCE 1453-1600

This era in history, produced a vigorous development of the arts and sciences inspired by the classical world. In a historical context this was the era establishing the necessary interface between medicine and the law. Thus, in 1507, there was the so called Code of Bamberg, ordering medical intervention and the hearing of expert opinion to clarify cases of homicide, infanticide and medical malpractices.

However, the start of the history of our discipline could be considered to be the *Constitutio Criminalis Carolina* which established where the intervention of doctors, surgeons and midwives was necessary. This would be in prosecuting cases of assault, murder, suicide of the mentally ill, births and abortions, infanticide, poisoning and medical errors.

The need for medical intervention performing a forensic function resulted in an era of writing on forensic medicine ensuring the foundation and growth of our science.

BAROQUE (1600-1740)

The first half of the seventeenth century is of paramount importance in the history of philosophy. Indeed, that is when, thanks to Galileo and Descartes, the foundation of modern theoretical and experimental science was developed.

In Spain, Juan Fragoso in 1601 published his *"Universal Surgery* in Alcala de Henares.

One of the four parts in which his work is divided comprises *'Statements that are to be made by surgeons about the diverse diseases and many causes of death'.*

The title is expressive enough to justify this author nicknamed *El Toledano, to* consider him the founder of the Spanish Legal Medicine but the major figure of this era is the Italian Paolo Zacchia (1584-1659), the father of Legal Medicine. Zacchia's work was extraordinary in its time and, even today, is usable in some respects.

A fundamental further step forward was made in 1637 when Descartes presents his 'Discourse on Method' defining a methodology for establishing fundamental truths in all areas of science.

THE AGE OF ENLIGHTENMENT (1740-1800).

This period produced enormous scientific progress fostered by both the organization of scientific work and by the emergence of scientific societies, facilitating exchanges and collaborations between scientists from different countries.

In Spain at this time there was relatively little development in the area of Forensic Medicine.

Fray Benito Jerónimo Feijoo between 1726 and 1740 published essays debunking common fallacies some relating to medico-legal issues asphyxia and death.

In 1796 Juan Fernandez del Valle published '*Forensic Surgery*', in three volumes, including the existing knowledge of Forensic Medicine of the time. This work was on a par with that of any of his contemporaries and in subsequent years was to be absorbed into Spanish Legal Medicine.

ROMANTICISM (1800-1848)

The development and expansion of Forensic Medicine in this period was cultivated by the boom in other branches of science, culminating in its inclusion in universities as an independent discipline.

In the field of toxicology special mention should be made of Matthew Joseph Bonaventure Orfila who published in 1814, a work titled *"Treatise on Poisons"*, that laid down the foundations of toxicology.

In 1831 Orfila made another great contribution to forensic medicine, in that year he published his *"Treatise on judicial exhumations and considerations on the physical changes of corpses decaying in the earth, water, latrines and manure"*. Any comment is superfluous.

The movement for incorporation of forensic medicine into the universities, started in Italy with the creation of the first chair, in 1789, occupied by Professor Ronchi, continuing in France (1794), Germany (1802.) and Austria (1805) ...

The first Spanish Chair was founded in 1843, and occupied by Professor Mata. This great expert issued a

"Treaty of Forensic Medicine", which collected together all the knowledge of legal medicine at the time.

Almost simultaneously the Chair in Barcelona was established, occupied by Professor Garcés Ferrer.

The final element which contributed to the growth and expansion of Forensic Medicine, was enacting clear legislation establishing its importance to society.

ERA OF REALISM AND NATURALISM (1848-1914)

Madrid's Forensic Medical Organization was established by a Royal Decree of 13 May 1862 this has evolved into the National Body that exists today and which finds its origin in the laws relating to health in 1855..

At the same time they also created the technical subsidiary bodies of the Administration of Justice which, as we shall see, are also of considerable value. The Central Laboratory of Forensic *Medicine,* now called National Institute of Toxicology was established in 1866.

In 1914 the Institute of Legal Medicine, Toxicology and Psychiatry in Central Spain was established subsequently becoming the current School of Legal Medicine, attached to the Complutense University Madrid. From it have come many experts in our field.

Finally, the publication of the Criminal Procedures Act of 1881 is also of great importance because it regulates many duties to be covered by medical examiners, or pathologists, in the field of criminal justice.

THE CURRENT ERA

I'll just mention three aspects that I consider of great interest to Spanish Forensic Medicine

One is the Constitutional Framework of 1978, developed from the Constitution of 1932 which has introduced some legislative changes having some obvious repercussions in the field of Forensic Medicine.

The second aspect is the enactment of the Judicial Power Organization Act of 6 July 1985, with successive amendments. It envisaged the creation of the Institutes of Legal Medicine. It is a way of trying to bring together and coordinate and rationalize the performance of the National Medical Examiners with the teaching and research activities developed in the Forensic Medicine Teaching Units. This is, moreover, the trend in most advanced countries in medico-legal organization.

The third important point, in direct relation with the previous one, is the final creation and specific regulation of the Institutes of Legal Medicine and the publication of new Regulation of Pathologists.

We are now approaching the end of both the history and the book. Some key figures of Legal Medicine of the immediate past, include: Lacasagne, Martin, Thoinot, Vibert, Dittrich, Richter, Strassman, Lochte, Ascarelli, Cevidalli, Sidney Smith, Bokarius, Lecha-Marzo, Alvarez De Toledo, Peset, Master. Piga etc ...

The Departments of Forensic Medicine in Spain and across Europe have been occupied mostly by outstanding disciples of the specialism amongst whom we could mention Muller, Ponsold, Prokoff, Berg, Piedelièvre, Simonin, Derobert , Roche, Michaux, Fazekas, Palmieri, Pellecrini, Royo-Villanova, Lopez Gomez, Perez De Petinto, Gisbert Calabuig, etc ...

Some of them, fortunately, continue to exercise their art; of others we treasure our memories, along with the extraordinary richness of their knowledge. I hope that my brief summary of the evolution of Legal Medicine has served to show that it has a strong historical scientific tradition. Now I have concluded.... really.

What I have tried to show was only a small part of what the Forensic Medicine is about. There is much,

much more. This you will find in the great writings of Legal Medicine or in the monographs and scientific articles published in various journals of our discipline. Also you will find more in the work and research of the Professorships and Training Units of Legal Medicine of the many Universities.

And you can see above all, every day, in different Spanish Courts members of the National Corps of Medical Examiners, to which I humbly belong, performing their duties.

If you now understand a little better the potential role of Forensic Medicine and its role assisting with the Administration of Justice, I am happy. I met one of the objectives sought when I started thinking about writing, which, incidentally, is coming to an end.

If you are thinking, or still think, that with the application of the knowledge and techniques of Legal Medicine a medical examiner who is given a fingernail can establish the cinematographic taste of the owner...sorry... my exposition has failed.

If you have enjoyed reading the various chapters, I'm glad; that was my hope. If it was boring; I apologise, but I congratulate you, because you had the stamina to reach the end. Finishing a book is the only way to say "that was pretty boring!"

At least that is what I have heard said by an inveterate reader, my mother.

10

Appendix: Who might have been there?

This chapter is completely new and is dedicated to one of the most important objectives of any criminal investigation; finding the perpetrator. Identification of the offender is a joint undertaking by a number of professionals with the main role being taken by the police investigators. Crime scene examination is carried out by forensic scientists and crime scene examiners applying a range of techniques but the forensic medical examiner, or pathologist, can also play an important role.

You will notice that in this part of the process, the forensic scientist may say much less; and in many cases, unfortunately cannot say anything ..... but we must not anticipate events.

Deciding on a title for this new chapter has not been easy. There were others which would have been more impressive, but would be misleading.

"Who did it?" For example, would have been nice.

But determining who committed a criminal act is not the job of the police, nor the forensic medical experts nor coroner. That is the job of the Judicial System, the magistrates, judges and members of the juries. Let them therefore decide whether the evidence is sufficient to bring a verdict of guilty. Such a title would also create false expectations; because at a crime scene there may be evidence of people who have never been there. There are many such possible scenarios; think of some and we'll see later if we agree.

In choosing the title for this final part of the book we are leaving open a number of possibilities. If at the scene of the crime, there are indications that an individual has been there, then it may be:

1. That the person has been there, but it has absolutely nothing to do with the offence.

2. That the individual in question has never been in the house of the deceased and there is a logical explanation for the presence of the forensic evidence.

3. That they are so involved in the incident that they have only failed to leave their signature, confession and identity card.

But, there are cases where despite calling on every possible forensic specialist there is no way to solve the case. Every police force has unsolved, pending, cases, which the police continue to investigate for many months or years...... Well, let's get on, that's enough of wasting time with dissertations on imponderables which get us nowhere. We must take the bull by the horns and accept things as they are.

In Chapter 3 we had a definition of identity: "Identity is the set of features that makes a person different from others and only equal to themself." Well, for the forensic scientist and the police to determine who could have been in a particular place they will use medical and biological data, but also much other unrelated information.

The search for evidence must be conducted initially on two fronts: the corpse and the scene.

A third front is opened up when they have obtained some indication of the suspects, and evidence may then be found in places associated with these suspects.

Well, we must pluck up courage and look at the corpse. The type of evidence that can be found on a body will be affected by two main factors: the type of crime committed and the precautions taken by the perpetrator. In addition there may be other factors if the victim has had the chance to defend themselves.

The case that we will consider is a rape, an example of sexual assault, associated with a high level of violence, and which has ended with the death of the victim.

Fingerprints, a fundamental method of identification, referred to elsewhere, may sometimes be detectable on the surface of a body. If they are going to be it is believed that the skin around the mouth, on the forearms, thighs or ankles is most amenable. Do not think that this is a simple or very successful process, but at least one should consider the possibility. If fingerprints are found it is of course easier if they are of a known offender than a 'first time offender'; although the value as evidence is the same.

Other types of evidence can be found in injuries to the body; let us see some examples._Within the broad group of skin injuries, bites, bruising and scratches are particularly important. From the first we find two types of evidence, the imprint of teeth left on the skin can be compared with the teeth of the suspects. For this, the bite mark must be photographed under carefully controlled conditions, then a sample bite from the suspect must be taken and the relevant comparison made.

The second type of evidence, to which we shall return later, is the saliva which has remained in the wound and its surroundings. From its genetic constituents the DNA profile of the person who has bitten the victim may be obtained.

Another aspect associated with the bites is where the victim has been able to defend themselves, and has bitten the assailant; there may even be traces of blood on the teeth.

So in this case there may be two types of evidence; from the blood, the genetic profile of the assailant may be obtained, and on the body of the assailant the bite mark may be compared with the imprint from the victim's teeth.

With the scratches the dimensions of the scratches that the nails of an aggressor have left on the body of the victim can serve to establish the approximate size of the hands. But what may be of greater value, as we have seen in more than one movie, is when the victim scratches the assailant. Then we will have the traces of the scratches on the body of the assailant and traces of blood or skin remaining under the nails on the body, from which we can obtain a DNA profile.

This explains why hands of corpses should be protected in plastic bags: so that no evidence is lost.

Another type of 'mark', perhaps less generally known to the public, are instrument marks. The English terminology for these marks is *toolmarks* and refers to any marks that an instrument or tool has left at a crime scene or, in this case, on a body.

There are many possible examples such as: the shape of the impact of a hammer or a wrench, the indentations of a knife, the characteristics of the toe of a boot, the initial engraved on a ring ... cheer up and think of some more examples.

As with bites and scratches these should be documented and recorded so that later photographic comparisons can be made with instruments which may have been involved. Also, if we are lucky, the instrument may have traces of the victim's blood or skin on it, which will serve to establish a definitive link.

In concluding the examination of corpses and identification of possible assailants let us look briefly at the biological evidence we can find on the deceased. I have already made a brief reference to evidence from bites; saliva, blood and DNA.

The study of such evidence, which I have covered in the chapter dedicated to the identification of the corpse, can be carried out on practically any biological material and provide valuable evidence of identity.

The introduction of DNA in criminal investigations has had two opposite effects. The first, favourable, that one can get a personal unambiguous identification, even if it does not always solve the case. The second unfortunate effect however, is a growing belief that without a DNA profile getting a conviction will be difficult.

But we should consider everything in its place; DNA is just one more tool to be used as part of the judicial process of the investigation of a crime. In no way should it replace a thorough investigation of all aspects. Because, as an example, the semen found on the corpse of a raped woman, does not necessarily come from the rapist.

I will tell you of a case in the United States with an unusual judicial procedure involving a serial rapist who has so far evaded arrest. The District Prosecutor, to avoid the statute of limitations, has pursued indictments of an individual contrary to the genetic profile of DNA found in the cases.

Well, you could say that what the forensic Medical Examiner can say has come to an end, because from now on other police experts are going to battle it out in court.

THE SCENE OF THE CRIME

As already indicated, the investigation of a crime is a set of procedures with the overall objective, as far as possible, of establishing the circumstances before, during and after the incident. One phase of it is investigating the crime scene. A fundamental premise is that, the place where a crime has been committed, the entirety, is in a continuously changing and transitory state.

Anyone entering a crime scene must be careful to avoid accelerating the changes or modifying unnecessarily the surroundings. The best way to achieve this is that those who know what they are doing get on with it, and those who do not, do nothing.

As the crime scene is a changing and unrepeatable entity the search for evidence by the Police and the Forensic Medical Examiners and Forensic Scientists, or Crime Scene Examiners, working closely together, should be:

CAREFUL AND UNRUSHED: Haste and impatience are always bad colleagues; we must however use the time well so that we do not leave too many loose ends to cause problems later.

EXTENSIVE: There must be no areas of the scene which have not been examined. If we use the English expression *the crime theatre,* common until the 1950s, it is easily understood that a theatre usually has a stage, but also has wings, orchestra pit, stalls, boxes, toilets etc. Similarly, the search for evidence should be done not only in the local area of the body, but must be extended as far as reason dictates.

THOROUGH: "No stone is to be left unturned". The important fingerprint may have been left on some page of a book. The traces of blood may be in the pocket of a pair of trousers kept in a cupboard. Again, sound reasoning should tell you where to end the search.

SUFFICIENT: To provide answers to most of the questions. The previous chapters have indicated the questions that we must try to answer. So we must search for the evidence which is going to give us answers to as many of those as possible. But, there is still scope for some imaginative thinking; think carefully where you might be able to find evidence; but imaginative thinking does not mean fantasy. It should be a process of logical reasoning forming a sound basis for further investigation. This need to think, when you're investigating, was expressed by Kongfuzi, usually known as Confucius, in the following maxim:

"Studying without thinking is futile. To think without studying is dangerous"

As already indicated the scene of a crime is a source of information and, if thoroughly investigated, will allow us to meet one or more of the following objectives:

DEFINING THE NATURE OF THE CRIME

The accurate characterization of the type of crime that has been committed is one of the primary purposes of the investigation. You must never forget that the precise details of any potentially criminal act may substantially affect the nature of any charges brought, and any subsequent penalties on conviction.

As an example: a person responsible for the death of another will be treated very differently depending on whether, during the trial, it can be shown it was an accident or it is established that it was the result of a deliberate act. In many cases, evidence found at the scene can be invaluable in defining the nature of the event, criminal or otherwise.

PROVIDING AVENUES OF FURTHER INVESTIGACION

This is one of the key elements; finding a fingerprint is of course of obvious significance. At other times, what may appear unimportant, traces of lipstick for example could be an identifiable lip print. Even the scent of a perfume can be of some use to the specialists.

ASSOCIATING THE CRIME SCENE OR VICTIM WITH ONE OR MORE INDIVIDUALS

Perhaps, as an example, to find at the scene some fibres that have some special characteristics which enable them to be matched with a garment in the possession of a suspect. Or associate them with some other person somehow connected to the victim.

TO CORROBORATE OR REFUTE THE ALIBI OF A SUSPECT

Continuing the example above someone may have indicated that an unrelated incident occurred that explained the presence of such fabric fibres at the scene. Obviously any observations documented by the expert should be corroborated by other aspects of the investigations.

IDENTIFY THE CULPRIT

This is of course, a main objective of any criminal investigation. In a case of strangulation perhaps we would like to find perfect, identifiable, fingerprints from the prime suspect on the victim's neck! This is the extreme example, but there are other less obvious, but equally conclusive possibilities.

EXONERATE THE INNOCENT

Sometimes it may happen that some circumstantial issues point to a particular person as the perpetrator of a crime. They may then declare their innocence and sometimes the contribution of the expert evidence is to exonerate the suspect's involvement in the events under investigation. Ultimately, it may be the courts that have to asses the evidence.

This means that, as one old and established Supreme Court ruling says *Dictum expertorum nunquam judicatam transit in rem,* that is, what experts say should not be considered as absolute but must be accepted or rejected for sound reasons.

ENTRY INTO THE CRIME SCENE: WHEN, WHO AND HOW.

In this brief section I will mention three very important aspects relating to the proper procedures for conducting the investigation which we must very carefully consider.

If, in the early stages, the wrong decisions are made, it can compromise the whole investigation.

WHEN

The first few hours that elapsed after the commission of a crime, are important. Therefore, we must not delay getting to our car. The passage of time increases the likelihood that evidence disappears or changes. So the sooner you get to examine the crime scene, the better the results will be. Notwithstanding that subsequently it may be necessary to continue the investigation for some time.

WHO

When a body is discovered if there is any possibility that the person is alive, the first intervention should of course be first aid. Therefore, the attendance of medical personnel is natural in these circumstances; but it is also important to record the exact position in which the body was found when the medical team arrived; to avoid subsequent misinterpretation.

Naturally, if the state of the body discovered leaves no doubts about its condition, odours, injuries, etc. it is not necessary to call the medical team.

The point, of course, is that the scene of a crime must only be attended by people who have some work to do there. Everyone else should stay away; this includes onlookers, family and friends, senior officers or anyone else not having a specific task to perform.

Sometimes you have to be very firm, but the reward is the reducing the chances of mistakes and the corruption or destruction of evidence. Establishing a police line and a secure perimeter is absolutely essential in all cases. This will keep out all those who are simply curious.

HOW

When many types of crime scenes are going to be investigated there should be documented procedures, or methods of work, for each. There cannot be just one, there may be three or four, so that there is one appropriate for each type of crime scene; open fields, in a domestic house, in large commercial premises etc.

The training of investigative teams in each of these scenarios is critical to achieving the objectives and as has been repeated earlier, time and dedication are essential.

WHAT CAN BE FOUND AT THE CRIME SCENE?

When talking about the crime scene usually we are thinking about a house or a room. But it must not be forgotten that this place may be a public road, a forest, etc. So the potential for finding evidence will be variable.

Briefly we can say that the materials which can provide further information to aid an investigation are

BLOOD, SEMEN, SALIVA AND OTHER FLUIDS OR TRACES OF BIOLOGICAL REMAINS

The study of these will be an important part of the investigation. They can be present in a variety of offences and their study is the basis of much forensic identification and permits the resolution of many cases.

The best thing, naturally, is to find a good spot of blood that does not belong to the victim and get the genetic profile. But now a genetic profile can very often be obtained from almost any type of biological material. Think where you can find traces of human genetic material, on:

A toothbrush.

A towel.

A bath sponge.

A lipstick.

A comb.

A razor.

The rim of a glass.

Chewing gum.

A lollipop or sweet.

Traces of dandruff found on the back of a chair

A wet-wipe.

A telephone mouthpiece.

A half-smoked cigarette.

All the aforementioned may retain sufficient genetic material so DNA extraction can be attempted..

And of saliva, football fans know that in the course of a game, players can discharge onto the ground litres of secretions. Does anyone remember that majestic spit of Arconada in a game they lost in Paris? The countless television replays allowed us to study in slow motion it's graceful swiveling motion that only lacked the backing of *The Blue Danube,* as in *2001 a Space Odyssey.*

If the murderer, or a thief, has the same nasty habit, he may be leaving you a wet track wherever he goes.

DOCUMENTS

Document Examination, is a specialist area of forensic science, although there are other organizations that have also developed a high levels of expertise in this area.

The physico-chemical aspects of paper or ink, and their age have been studied and there are techniques to establish whether there have been additions or alterations to writing. It is also possible to see if two documents have been produced by the same person, and so on. Such handwriting comparison can make decisive contributions.

On the other hand, applying graphological techniques, may suggest the psychological state of a writer. As you can imagine, this is especially important for suicide notes or for cases involving anonymous letters.

FIBERS

The analysis of fibers is another very specialized field of investigation. Traces of fabric fibres may be found on a corpse or furniture or other belongings at a scene.

It is also possible that, for example, the vehicle of a suspect may contain some fibers from the clothing of the deceased. Naturally, these are particularly valuable when the suspect cannot give a satisfactory innocent explanation for why they are there.

FRICTION RIDGE DETAILS

The study of ridge detail forms a significant contribution to identification of individuals.

FINGERPRINTS

If I remember correctly, this is the third time that I mention them. So we have already commented on their high value for identification and here we will only clarify a few things. The first is that, at the scene of a crime, one can find fingerprints in very different forms.

Sometimes there may be many, clear, obvious and visible fingerprints. Other times however there may be only a few fragments invisible to the naked eye. Of course a fingerprint identification does not necessarily imply responsibility for a crime. As always, they must be considered in the overall context of the investigation.

Remember that this chapter is not called *"Who was there?"* We have to try to answer a different question; because, for example, the fingerprints of a person may appear on the hammer that was used to strike the head of the victim. But of course that does not necessarily mean that the owner of the fingerprints has been at the crime scene?

HAND AND FOOT PRINTS

The prints of hands and feet can have a dual function. Fingerprints have been used by police for a long time for identification of individuals and for many years there have been fingerprint databases for this purpose. Take a look at your hands, please, and you will see you also have lines, wrinkles, etc. these are also very characteristic

The prints of bare feet can also be used for identification, in fact, taking the prints of the soles of the feet of newborn babies is one method to avoid mistakes, still used in many hospitals. It is now being replaced by taking a blood sample to compare the DNA with the parent.

The second value of the handprints and bare feet is more general information. Apart from a few anomalies and exceptions, the latter, you know, are those that prove the rule, there is proportionality between the size of the limbs and the rest of the body. Thus, one can start looking for suspects that have certain physical attributes.

SHOEPRINTS

If you are interested go to your cupboard and take out one of your trainer shoes. On one of mine I read: *"43, Uniroyal, Made in Spain, A-03-009149";* it may also have distinctive wear patterns. Well, all that can be printed on the floor. That is pretty useful for the police, don't you think?

Other information can be obtained by specialized study of footwear impressions; if they walked or ran, whether they were on tiptoe at some point, the length of the legs, if they were carrying a substantial load, when on soft ground.

You may even be able to say something about the sex of those who have left the track.

Mens' or womens' shoes can be dissimilar but may mislead; but the gait of men and women are different. Under ideal conditions, by studying the impressions and gait, forensic examination may answer this question.

From the footwear impressions, apart from information on the identity of the wearer, crystallographic and physical-chemical analysis of soil in the prints can provide information on where they may have been.

Similarly, in cases where a body is found in a forest or open space, analysis of soil traces from the clothes and comparison with where the body is found may show discrepancies which indicate that the body has been moved.

LIP PRINTS

That telltale print that so often we have seen in ads for cosmetics, may be more or less sexy, but also has evidential value to the police. Like other parts of our body, the lips have unique features that leave their characteristics; and they can be identified as belonging to an individual.

As an example of a real case: a person enters a bank and steals some cash. Security cameras record the scene.

When the thief, with long blond hair, in this case, tried to go out into the street, the wrong way they hit their face against the glass and curse. The police investigation implicated a man; but the imprint of lips found on the glass was identified as belonging to a woman.

And do not think that the 'permanent' lipstick, those that 'leave no trace', cannot be detected. Liprints are left and are detectable.

Ana Castelló, Mercedes Alvarez, Marcos Miquel and this author, have carried out carefully studies of these. The difference in the residues from traditional cosmetics is that they are not visible with the naked eye. There is therefore a need to use something to develop them as with fingerprints.

EAR PRINTS

Yes, ladies and gentlemen, your ears are also very distinctive and particular to the individual. And this is no modern idea, since in the latter part of the eighteenth century there are references to the usefulness of the ears as a means of identification.

This is a good time to stop reading. Look at some childrens' ears, and their parents. Look for similarities and differences.

Ear prints often appear in very specific locations: doors, windows, walls ... where you want to hear what's happening on the other side or if you want to check somewhere they want to break in, that nobody is at home. They are revealed by the same techniques used for fingerprints.

The final step is to compare the imprint found with the suspect's. So we have another method to be used in an investigation.

According to legend and films the Wild West must have had the sands thick with the impressions of ears of Indians or cowboys listening for horses hooves. I promise I will try not to exercise my sense of humour any more.

So we have finished the study of prints, only two or three other things to say about the scene of a crime.

GARBAGE

The garbage cans are, it is well known, real 'black box recorders' of the homes from which they come. By the analysis of the household waste, you can find out much about the behaviour and habits of its inhabitants and this can also prove useful in criminal investigations.

You can assess the dehydration of food remains, to relate it to the time of death. Also, for similar purposes, you may try to establish the composition of foods eaten in the last few hours.

Also, the bar codes that appear on virtually all packaging, give information on their origin. In that way can we know, approximately, when they were acquired and in the most favourable circumstances, get some help with who may have acquired them.

As a final example, those containers and wrappers are also excellent media for carrying other evidential traces. Fingerprints or marks left by the teeth of a person perhaps in an apple.

TAPED VOICES AND NOISES

Of course these may be evidence of vital importance. Voices recorded on tape or in an answering machine have individual personal characteristics which can be analyzed.

This is a technique performed by the police in some special laboratories; in Spain a system called 'Locupol' has been developed for the creation of a database of voice recordings.

The analysis of background noises or music on recordings can also help research in certain aspects concerning location etc.

Remember that it was the sound of bells, which allowed an accomplice of Bin Laden to be located in the fall of 2001.

OTHER

As I have shown and repeated; my indication that a crime scene is a fund of data has not been made lightly. There are many possible things to examine and analyze which may help an investigation.

For example, the finding of a contact lens in the car of someone suspected of rape and murder.

A body was found in a field and the forensic medical examination report indicated that only one contact lens was in place. The optical properties and composition of this lens were measured in collaboration with the optician that made the lenses. Fragments of a contact lens were found in the vehicle of a suspect and we established that it was the lens missing from corpse. The suspect could not give a clear explanation about how he got there that lens.

Condoms are also objects that should be investigated and can prove very informative. Of course the most obvious is their source of material for DNA. But there's more.

You can study the composition of the rubber used in its manufacture. You can also find out the characteristics of the lubricants used to facilitate its use, the type of spermicide, and other treatment and products used in manufacture. With all that, you can locate the manufacturer; as in the case of paints, plastics and glass, there are always variations in the composition. The last final step is to establish where the manufacturer retails its products. You may have a place to start your search.

Now this Appendix ends; it could cover more but I am sure you readers will think of other ways to find the murderer.

Back to work!

Good Luck!

NOTES

NOTES

NOTES